Praise for *Craniosynostosis*

"This is one of the most comprehensive and educational books on the subject of craniosynostosis. I congratulate Dr. Barta and the team at Gillette Children's for putting together a thorough, detailed, and well-written book. It covers all aspects of craniosynostosis and plagiocephaly, and it is a valuable resource for providers and patients and their families. The educational material that is elegantly presented provides patients and their families with the information they need to make an informed decision, and it highlights the unique and holistic treatment approach followed by the experts at Gillette Children's."

WALEED GIBREEL, Pediatric Plastic and Craniofacial Surgeon, Mayo Clinic, Rochester, Minnesota

"I found the book very educational and easy to read. I think it will help many new families beginning the craniosynostosis journey. Very well written!"

SHELBY DAVIDSON, Parent of child with sagittal craniosynostosis, Seattle, Washington

"I had the pleasure of reading Craniosynostosis, *authored by health care providers Ruth Barta, MD, and Cheryl Tveit, RN, with parent Heather Comstock. This is a remarkably comprehensive review of all things related to craniosynostosis and is a terrific source of information for parents and families of infants and children affected by this rare and complex condition. It leaves no stone unturned. I hope it brings some level of comfort to parents and patients dealing with the challenges of craniosynostosis."*

CHRISTOPHER R. FORREST, Medical Director, SickKids Craniofacial Program, Toronto; Professor, Division of Plastic, Reconstructive and Aesthetic Surgery, University of Toronto

"This is an excellent and informative book that is both clear and factual. It serves as a valuable resource for families, providing them with essential knowledge about craniosynostosis and empowering them to engage confidently with medical and health professionals. The personal stories included offer hope and reassurance, reminding families that they are not alone in their journey. This is the book I wish I had when my son was diagnosed with sagittal craniosynostosis in 2019."

ELAINE L. KINSELLA, Parent; Chartered Psychologist and Associate Professor in Psychology, University of Limerick, Ireland

"Receiving a diagnosis of craniosynostosis can be scary; it's a condition most parents have never heard of. This book is the perfect starting point for anyone looking to understand the basics and to help them navigate the treatment options available as best practices in craniofacial surgery continue to evolve."

JEFFREY FEARON, Director Craniofacial Center, Dallas, Texas; President Emeritus of the American Society of Craniofacial Surgeons and the Texas Society of Plastic Surgeons

T0344671

"This book provides an insightful exploration into the complexities of craniosynostosis, a condition where the bones in an infant's skull fuse prematurely. Through a blend of personal narrative and scientific research, it offers a comprehensive understanding of the condition's causes, symptoms, and treatment options. What sets this book apart is its compassionate portrayal of families affected by craniosynostosis. By sharing their stories, the authors shed light on the emotional challenges they face, from diagnosis to treatment decisions. Additionally, the book delves into the latest medical advancements, offering hope to families navigating this complex problem. It serves as an informative resource for those seeking knowledge about the condition; its real strength lies in its ability to inspire empathy and solidarity among readers."

EMMA CORDES, Assistant Professor, Indiana University Department of Surgery, Division of Plastic Surgery; Director of Cleft and Craniofacial Program; Director of Global Surgery Program

"Craniosynostosis will be a valuable resource, especially for parents who are just learning of their child's diagnosis. The detailed explanation of the condition, the pronunciation of words, and the definitions are all beneficial to the reader in providing information all in one place—my favorite aspect. Incorporating personal stories gives a sense of reality, as well as comfort and reassurance often sought by those affected by craniosynostosis. I firmly believe this book will help educate and bring further awareness to the condition."

LINDSAY WALKER, Parent of a child with nonsyndromic craniosynostosis, West Virginia

"This is a great reference book for all things craniosynostosis. It is appropriate for medical professionals as well as parents and caregivers who want to dig deeper into what they might anticipate for their child—not only in the early period of surgery but also beyond. The book is well designed and organized in such a way that the reader can more specifically find what they need. The personal stories and photographs so graciously shared by the families speak to how those having a child with craniosynostosis are affected in a way that we as providers are unable to fully comprehend. We know how to take care of these kids; families know what it is like to live it."

CHERYL HOLIHAN, Pediatric Nurse Practitioner Otolaryngology, University of Texas Southwestern, Dallas; Volunteer, Children's Surgery International

"As parents of a child with metopic CS we are certain this book will be a valuable resource to all. It provides both tactical information and human experiences through all phases of CS, from recognition to diagnosis, surgery and recovery, research, and beyond. We are so grateful for the continued research and education Gillette Children's is leading."

STACY AND ANDREW STUECK, Parents of child with metopic CS, Minnesota

CRANIOSYNOSTOSIS

CRANIOSYNOSTOSIS

Understanding and
managing the condition:
A practical guide
for families

Ruth J. Barta, MD
Cheryl Tveit, RN, MSN, CNML
Heather Comstock, Parent

Edited by
Lily Collison, MA, MSc
Elizabeth R. Boyer, PhD
Martin Lacey, MD
Tom F. Novacheck, MD
GILLETTE CHILDREN'S

Gillette Children's Healthcare Press
200 University Avenue East
St Paul, MN 55101
www.GilletteChildrensHealthcarePress.org
HealthcarePress@gillettechildrens.com

ISBN 978-1-952181-09-2 (paperback)
ISBN 978-1-952181-10-8 (e-book)
LIBRARY OF CONGRESS CONTROL NUMBER 2024941533

COPYEDITING BY Ruth Wilson
ORIGINAL ILLUSTRATIONS BY Olwyn Roche
COVER AND INTERIOR DESIGN BY Jazmin Welch
PROOFREADING BY Ruth Wilson
INDEX BY Audrey McClellan

Printed by Hobbs the Printers Ltd, Totton, Hampshire, UK

For information about distribution or special discounts for bulk purchases,
please contact:
Mac Keith Press
2nd Floor, Rankin Building
139-143 Bermondsey Street
London, SE1 3UW
www.mackeith.co.uk
admin@mackeith.co.uk

The views and opinions expressed herein are those of the authors and
Gillette Children's Healthcare Press and do not necessarily represent those
of Mac Keith Press.

To individuals and families whose lives are affected by these conditions, to professionals who serve our community, and to all clinicians and researchers who push the knowledge base forward, we hope the books in this Healthcare Series serve you very well.

All proceeds from the books in this series at Gillette Children's go to research.

All information contained in this book is for educational purposes only. For specific medical advice and treatment, please consult a qualified health care professional. The information in this book is not intended as a substitute for consultation with your health care professional.

Contents

Authors and Editors

Ruth J. Barta, MD, Craniofacial and Pediatric Plastic Surgeon, Gillette Children's

Cheryl Tveit, RN, MSN, CNML, Principal Writer, Gillette Children's Healthcare Press

Heather Comstock, Parent

Lily Collison, MA, MSc, Program Director, Gillette Children's Healthcare Press

Elizabeth R. Boyer, PhD, Clinical Scientist, Gillette Children's

Martin Lacey, MD, Craniofacial and Plastic Surgeon Emeritus, Gillette Children's

Tom F. Novacheck, MD, Medical Director of Integrated Care Services, Gillette Children's; Professor of Orthopedics, University of Minnesota; and Past President, American Academy for Cerebral Palsy and Developmental Medicine

Series Foreword

You hold in your hands one book in the Gillette Children's Healthcare Series. This series was inspired by multiple factors.

It started with Lily Collison writing the first book in the series, *Spastic Diplegia–Bilateral Cerebral Palsy*. Lily has a background in medical science and is the parent of a now adult son who has spastic diplegia. Lily was convincing at the time about the value of such a book, and with the publication of that book in 2020, Gillette Children's became one of the first children's hospitals in the world to set up its own publishing arm—Gillette Children's Healthcare Press. *Spastic Diplegia–Bilateral Cerebral Palsy* received very positive reviews from both families and professionals and achieved strong sales. Unsolicited requests came in from diverse organizations across the globe for translation rights, and feedback from families told us there was a demand for books relevant to other conditions.

We listened.

We were convinced of the value of expanding from one book into a series to reflect Gillette Children's strong commitment to worldwide education. In 2021, Lily joined the press as Program Director, and very quickly, Gillette Children's formed teams to write the Healthcare Series. The series includes, in order of publication:

- *Craniosynostosis*
- *Idiopathic Scoliosis*
- *Spastic Hemiplegia—Unilateral Cerebral Palsy*
- *Spastic Quadriplegia—Bilateral Cerebral Palsy*
- *Spastic Diplegia—Bilateral Cerebral Palsy, second edition*
- *Epilepsy*
- *Spina Bifida*
- *Osteogenesis Imperfecta*
- *Scoliosis—Congenital, Neuromuscular, Syndromic, and Other Causes*

The books address each condition detailing both the medical and human story.

Mac Keith Press, long-time publisher of books on disability and the journal *Developmental Medicine and Child Neurology,* is co-publishing this series with Gillette Children's Healthcare Press.

Families and professionals working well together is key to best management of any condition. The parent is the expert of their child while the professional is the expert of the condition. These books underscore the importance of that family and professional partnership. For each title in the series, medical professionals at Gillette Children's have led the writing, and families contributed the lived experience.

These books have been written in the United States with an international lens and citing international research. However, there isn't always strong evidence to create consensus in medicine, so others may take a different view.

We hope you find the book you hold in your hands to be of great value. We collectively strive to optimize outcomes for children, adolescents, and adults living with these childhood-acquired and largely lifelong conditions.

Dr. Tom F. Novacheck

Series Introduction

The Healthcare Series seeks to optimize outcomes for those who live with childhood-acquired physical and/or neurological conditions. The conditions addressed in this series of books are complex and often have many associated challenges. Although the books focus on the biomedical aspects of each condition, we endeavor to address each condition as holistically as possible. Since the majority of people with these conditions have them for life, the life course is addressed including transition and aging issues.

Who are these books for?

These books are written for an international audience. They are primarily written for parents of young children, but also for adolescents and adults who have the condition. They are written for members of multidisciplinary teams and researchers. Finally, they are written for others, including extended family members, teachers, and students taking courses in the fields of medicine, allied health care, and education.

A worldview

The books in the series focus on evidence-based best practice, which we acknowledge is not available everywhere. It is mostly available in high-income countries (at least in urban areas, though even there, not always), but many families live away from centers of good care.

We also acknowledge that the majority of people with disabilities live in low- and middle-income countries. Improving the lives of all those with disabilities across the globe is an important goal. Developing scalable, affordable interventions is a crucial step toward achieving this. Nonetheless, the best interventions will fail if we do not first address the social determinants of health—the economic, social, and environmental conditions in which people live that shape their overall health and well-being.

No family reading these books should ever feel they have failed their child. We all struggle to do our best for our children within the limitations of our various resources and situations. Indeed, the advocacy role these books may play may help families and professionals lobby in unison for best care.

International Classification of Functioning, Disability and Health

The writing of the series of books has been informed by the International Classification of Functioning, Disability and Health (ICF).[1] The framework explains the impact of a health condition at different levels and how those levels are interconnected. It tells us to look at the full picture—to look at the person with a disability in their life situation.

The framework shows that every human being can experience a decrease in health and thereby experience some disability. It is not something that happens only to a minority of people. The ICF thus "mainstreams" disability and recognizes it as a widespread human experience.

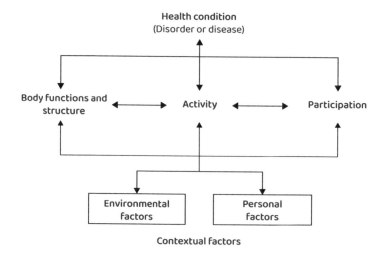

International Classification of Functioning, Disability and Health (ICF). Reproduced with kind permission from WHO.

In health care, there has been a shift away from focusing almost exclusively on correcting issues that cause the individual's functional problems to focusing also on the individual's activity and participation. These books embrace maximizing participation for all people living with disability.

The family

For simplicity, throughout the series we refer to "parents" and "children"; we acknowledge, however, that family structures vary. "Parent" is used as a generic term that includes grandparents, relatives, and carers (caregivers) who are raising a child. Throughout the series, we refer to male and female as the biologic sex assigned at birth. We acknowledge that this does not equate to gender identity or sexual orientation, and we respect the individuality of each person. Throughout the series we have included both "person with disability" and "disabled person," recognizing that both terms are used.

Caring for a child with a disability can be challenging and overwhelming. Having a strong social support system in place can make a difference. For the parent, balancing the needs of the child with a disability with the needs of siblings—while also meeting employment demands, nurturing a relationship with a significant other, and caring for aging parents—can sometimes feel like an enormous juggling act. Siblings may feel neglected or overlooked because of the increased attention given to the disabled child. It is crucial for parents to allocate time and resources to ensure that siblings feel valued and included in the family dynamics. Engaging siblings in the care and support of the disabled child can help foster a sense of unity and empathy within the family.

A particular challenge for a child and adolescent who has a disability, and their parent, is balancing school attendance (for both academic and social purposes) with clinical appointments and surgery. Appointments outside of school hours are encouraged. School is important because the cognitive and social abilities developed there help maximize employment opportunities when employment is a realistic goal. Indeed, technology has eliminated barriers and created opportunities that did not exist even 10 years ago.

Parents also need to find a way to prioritize self-care. Neglecting their own well-being can have detrimental effects on their mental and physical health. Think of the safety advice on an airplane: you are told that you must put on your own oxygen mask before putting on your child's. It's the same when caring for a child with a disability; parents need to take care of themselves in order to effectively care for their child *and* family. Friends, support groups, or mental health professionals can provide an outlet for parents to express their emotions, gain valuable insights, and find solace in knowing that they are not alone in their journey.

Last words

This series of books seeks to be an invaluable educational resource. All proceeds from the series at Gillette Children's go to research.

Chapter 1

Craniosynostosis

Introduction

Growth is never by mere chance;
it is the result of forces working together.

J.C. Penney

If you are reading this as a parent of a child recently diagnosed with craniosynostosis, this term may be new to you. It is pronounced "kray-nee-o-sin-os-TOE-sis" (the capitals indicate emphasis on that syllable). Craniosynostosis (CS) is a condition where the bones of the skull fuse together too early. While CS may not be noticed immediately by parents or medical professionals, it is a condition present from birth; therefore, it is known as a congenital condition.

Congenital CS is also referred to as primary CS.[*] It is relatively uncommon, occurring in 1 in 2,500 births.[3] In most cases, surgery in the first year of life will effectively correct it and those affected can expect a typical life (this is *nonsyndromic* CS). For a minority, CS is part of a syndrome, which is a lifelong condition (this is *syndromic* CS).

---

[*] Another type of CS, secondary CS, develops secondary to atypical brain development or other medical conditions; it is uncommon and is not included in this book.[2]

The term "craniosynostosis" comes from "cranio," meaning cranium (skull); "syn," meaning together; "ost," meaning bone; and "osis," meaning condition.

The medical definition of CS is:

> *The premature, pathologic fusion of one or more cranial sutures leading to an abnormal cranial shape that can subsequently result in facial deformities and increased intracranial pressure.*[4]

Table 1.1.1 further explains the terms used in the definition of CS.

Table 1.1.1 Terms in the definition of CS

TERM	EXPLANATION
Abnormal	Deviating from the typical expectation; atypical
Cranial	Relating to the skull
Deformities	Malformations or misshapen parts of the body
Facial	Referring to something affecting or concerning the face
Fusion	The process of joining two or more things together to form one
Intracranial pressure	The measure of pressure inside the skull
Pathologic	Referring to the involvement, cause, or nature of a condition
Premature	Referring to something occurring too early or before the usual or proper time
Suture	An immovable junction between two bones; cranial sutures are fibrous joints that connect the bones of the skull (not to be confused with surgical stitches, which are also called sutures)

The early fusion of the cranial sutures in CS causes the skull and face to become misshapen and may lead to further complications if not treated. Many of these skull shapes and sutures were first described centuries ago. Figure 1.1.1 shows early drawings of skull shapes and sutures.

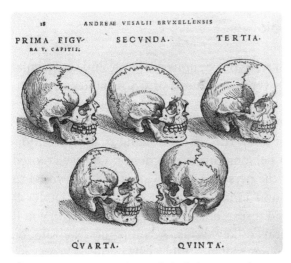

Figure 1.1.1 Early drawings of skull shapes and sutures (about 1543). Reproduced with kind permission from Syndromic craniosynostosis: from history to hydrogen bonds, by Cunningham et al. (2007) in *Orthod Craniofacial Res*, 10, 67-81.

The term "craniosynostosis" was first used by Otto in 1830. As early as 1851, Rudolph Virchow, a German physician, explained that a skull can expand evenly only when the sutures are appropriately open on all sides of the skull.[5] When a suture fuses prematurely, other areas in the skull compensate and get pushed apart to accommodate brain growth. This theory became known as Virchow's law, and it allows us to predict the skull shape based on the fused sutures.[6] Specifically, Virchow's law states:

> *When premature fusion of the cranial vault* occurs there is an inhibition of the normal growth of the skull in a direction perpendicular to the suture which is fused, which gives a compensatory growth in a direction parallel to the fused suture.*[8]

The atypical head shape in CS is caused by unequal *internal* forces on the skull (the fused sutures), but *external* forces may also contribute to an atypical head shape. When external forces are involved, it's called "deformational plagiocephaly" (pronounced as plag-jee-oh-sef-uh-lee) and is sometimes confused with CS. Indeed, deformational plagiocephaly may simultaneously occur with CS, but it is *not* CS. Deformational plagiocephaly is described in Chapter 5.

---

* The cranial vault is the space that encases and protects the brain.[7]

How to read this book

This book is relevant to both types of CS: nonsyndromic and syndromic. This chapter addresses the overall condition of CS. Chapters 2 and 6 are specific to nonsyndromic craniosynostosis, and Chapters 3 and 7 are specific to syndromic craniosynostosis. The remaining Chapters—4, 5, 8, and 9—will be of interest to all readers. Throughout, medical information is interspersed with personal lived experience. Orange-colored boxes are used to highlight the personal story. Chapter 8 is devoted to vignettes from individuals and families around the globe. Chapter 9 addresses further reading and research. At the back of this book, you'll find a glossary with definitions of key terms. A companion website for this book is available at www.GilletteChildrensHealthcarePress.org. This website contains several resources, including **Useful web resources** (QR code below).

USEFUL WEB RESOURCES

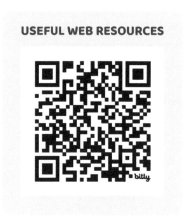

My name is Heather, and I have been married to my husband, Jason, for almost 20 years. We live in the suburbs of Saint Paul, Minnesota. We have two boys and a girl, each two years apart. Our middle child, Keegan, was born with craniosynostosis.

I have worked at a Level 1 trauma center[*] for the last 15 years as a physician assistant[†] and thoroughly enjoy helping patients and their families achieve the best outcomes with their health. Once the term "craniosynostosis" came into our lives, and our son went through his cranio journey, we developed a newfound passion: to spread craniosynostosis awareness.

Keegan was born on a Saturday, late in the evening, with temperatures outside below freezing. Our firstborn son was at home with my parents, anxiously awaiting news of his baby brother's arrival. Labor progressed similarly to my first labor until it was time to push. We anticipated a speedy delivery, but it took more pushing than expected. Keegan's heartbeat would go down with contractions, which was a bit worrisome. They decided to use a vacuum to facilitate birth, which was used for just a minute because Keegan then decided to enter the world.

When he came out, the doctor found the umbilical cord was wrapped around his neck twice. We were so relieved when we heard him cry for the first time. I recall my husband seeing him first and making a comment about having some buggy eyes. I felt slightly concerned and thought that was an odd thing to say, but by the time I was able to meet him, he could not have been more perfect. He had big, beautiful eyes that were a very deep, slate-colored blue. He stole our hearts from that moment. We did notice he had a mark on the top of his head in the shape of a heart, likely caused by bruising during delivery. At the time, we thought it was sweet. Little did we know how much it would actually come to mean to us.

---

* In the US, a hospital that is capable of providing total care to patients through all aspects of a traumatic injury, as designated by the American Trauma Society.[9]

† A medical professional licensed to practice medicine in every specialty and setting in the United States and other jurisdictions. The training is modeled after medical school education, with a generalized focus, allowing them to care for all ages.[10] Physician assistants require graduate schooling and have greater medical privileges (e.g., diagnosing, prescribing) than nurses and work alongside a supervising physician.

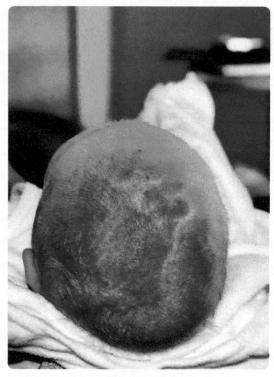

Keegan, just after birth.

We first heard the term "craniosynostosis" when we brought Keegan in for his two-week well-child visit.* It was a new term for my husband. If I had learned about craniosynostosis in physician assistant school, it was just a mention—at most—in the pediatrics section, not enough to even trigger a memory of the term.

---

* In the US, well-child visits are regular appointments with medical professionals (typically as recommended by the American Academy of Pediatrics: three to five days after birth, then several times over the first 30 months, and then annually until adulthood). They often coincide with vaccination schedules and include growth and development tracking and monitoring.[11] These visits may be done in other countries, too, but may be known by other names and may occur with different timing.

Typical brain and skull development

The only reason for time is so that everything doesn't happen at once.

Albert Einstein

To understand CS, it is important to have a good understanding of brain and skull development. That includes understanding certain terms that are used throughout this book when referring to areas of the body. Table 1.2.1 lists directional terms used in anatomy, which are used specifically in this section (and generally throughout the book). (See the Glossary for a full list of terms used in this book.)

Table 1.2.1 Terms used to describe anatomical direction

TERM	EXPLANATION	VIEW
Anterior	Near the front, or front side	Front
Lateral	Away from the midline (or middle of the body), referring to the side	Side
Posterior	Near the back, or back side	Back
Superior	Above or looking down from above	Top

Embryonic and fetal skull development

An embryo is a developing human from conception up to the end of the eighth week after conception—referred to as the embryonic period. A fetus is a developing human from the eighth week after conception to birth.[12] "Prenatal" refers to the period before birth, and "perinatal" to the period around the time of birth.[13,14]

The brain and skull start to develop during the embryonic period. The cranial bones, or the skull bones, form approximately six to eight weeks after conception and the cranial sutures between 15 and 18 weeks.[12,15,16] Figure 1.2.1 shows the cranial bones in a fetus 12 weeks after conception. The gaps between the cranial bones are the areas where the cranial sutures will develop.

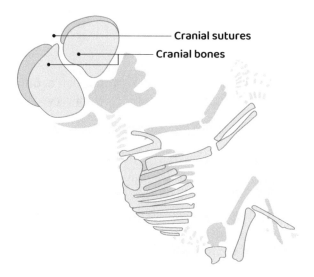

Cranial sutures
Cranial bones

Figure 1.2.1 Fetal skeleton 12 weeks after conception.

a) Brain and skull development

At birth, the newborn* skull is made up of separate bones that are not yet fused. This allows for easier passage through the birth canal and rapid brain growth after birth. The skull protects the brain during this growth period—the brain triples in size by the time the child reaches one year of age.[5,7] This brain growth drives the growth of the skull, especially in the first few years of life. As the brain expands, it pushes the skull bones apart along the sutures, and the body creates and lays down new bone in between,[18] eventually forming the mature skull. With CS, this process is disrupted and the sutures fuse too early, which may negatively impact brain development if left untreated.

b) Cranial bones

There are many bones in the human skull, together called the cranial bones. The largest of the cranial bones make up the cranial vault, which is the space that encases and protects the brain.[7]

Figure 1.2.2 shows the newborn skull from the side (lateral view) and the top (superior view). The two frontal bones (teal) are on the skull's front (anterior); the two parietal bones (orange) are on the upper sides of the skull; the temporal bones (pink) are on the lower sides, so they are not visible in the superior view; and the occipital bone (purple) is at the back (posterior).

---

* A newborn is a child from birth to four weeks of age; an infant is a child from birth to one year of age.[17]

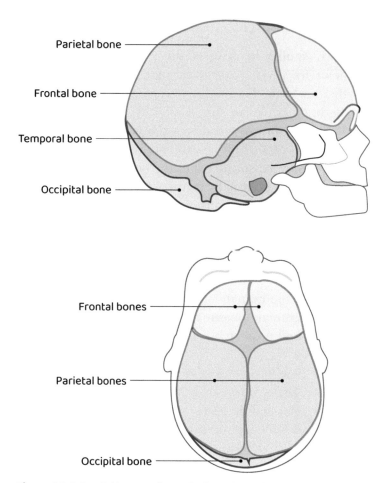

Parietal bone

Frontal bone

Temporal bone

Occipital bone

Frontal bones

Parietal bones

Occipital bone

Figure 1.2.2 Cranial bones of a typical newborn: lateral view (top); superior view (bottom).

The cranial bones protect the brain and other structures in the skull. In Figure 1.2.3, notice the rounded frontal bones and orbital sockets (the openings for the eyes in the skull). One key function of the frontal bones is to protect the eyes. The supraorbital rim (the upper edge of the orbital socket) of each eye is formed by the frontal bone, and this design offers protection by creating brow bones that provide a cover over the eye-balls. In some forms of CS, this protective feature can be lost, leaving the eyes susceptible to injury.

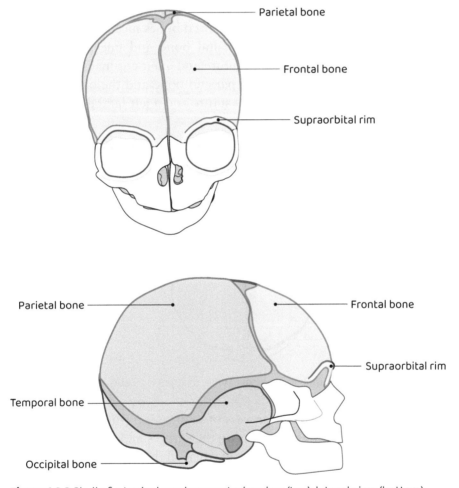

Figure 1.2.3 Skull of a typical newborn: anterior view (top); lateral view (bottom).

c) Cranial sutures

Cranial sutures are the fibrous joints that connect the bones of the skull. These are divided into major and minor sutures. While the minor sutures can also fuse prematurely, they rarely need surgical correction and are, therefore, not described here.

The major sutures are shown in Figure 1.2.4:

- **Sagittal suture:** Where the two parietal bones meet
- **Metopic suture:** Where the two frontal bones meet
- **Coronal suture:** Where one frontal bone and one parietal bone meet; there is a right coronal suture and a left coronal suture
- **Lambdoid suture:** Where one parietal bone and the occipital bone meet; there is a right lambdoid suture and a left lambdoid suture

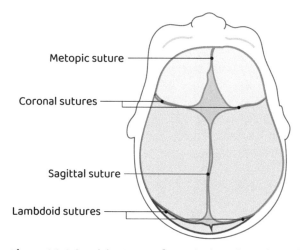

Figure 1.2.4 Cranial sutures of a typical newborn (superior view).

Suture fusion is the gradual process of ossification (turning into bone) of the fibrous material that makes up the sutures and the bones joining together. A suture is considered fused when all that remains is a thin line where the bones are joined. Figure 1.2.5 shows two views of a newborn skull, with open sutures, and two views of an adult skull, with fused sutures, for comparison.

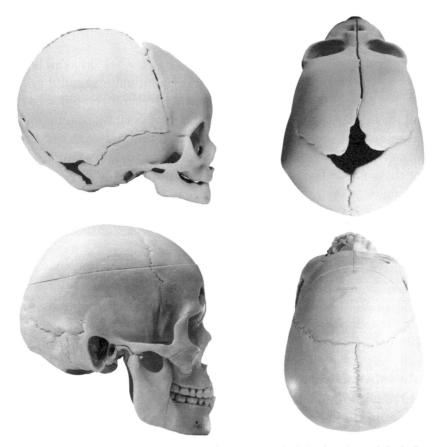

Figure 1.2.5 Lateral and superior views of a newborn skull (top) and an adult skull (bottom).

The sutures generally fuse in order from front to back (anterior to posterior) and from the sides to the midline.[19]

- The metopic suture is the first suture to fuse and the only major suture to normally close in infancy. It sometimes starts fusing as early as 3 months of age and is typically completely fused by 9 to 12 months of age.[5,7,20]
- The sagittal, coronal, and lambdoid sutures begin fusing between the ages of 20 and 29 years.[5,21]

The premature fusion of these sutures in newborns or infants, as occurs with CS, can impact head shape and other aspects of health if left untreated, especially if more than one suture is involved.

d) Cranial fontanels

Cranial fontanels are the areas where the "corners" of the skull bones meet. You can feel them in newborns and young infants, and they are sometimes called "the soft spot" because they feel soft compared to the rest of the head. As the infant grows, the fontanels close from the edges to the middle, as the body creates new bone, eventually covering them completely. It's important to note that the disappearance of fontanels is not the same as fusion of the bones or suture fusion. However, certain changes to the fontanels, such as persistent bulging or an atypical shape, may raise concern.[22]

There are several fontanels in the newborn skull. Figure 1.2.6 shows the two main ones.

- The anterior fontanel is toward the front of the head and is the largest fontanel, making it easy to find. It is at the junction of the coronal, metopic, and sagittal sutures. The anterior fontanel typically fills in between 12 and 18 months.[22,23]
- The smaller posterior fontanel is toward the back of the head. It is at the junction of the lambdoid and sagittal sutures. This fontanel typically fills in by approximately two months of age.[23]

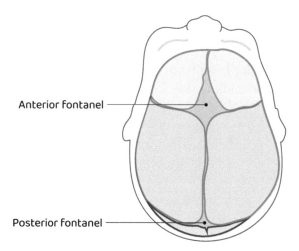

Anterior fontanel

Posterior fontanel

Figure 1.2.6 Cranial fontanels of a typical newborn (superior view).

I had two miscarriages before our first child was born. Both were early in the pregnancy. After our first child was born, we became pregnant again and I was cautiously optimistic, but I also was mentally preparing for another miscarriage. The pregnancy did indeed last, without any prenatal concerns. Every checkup and ultrasound showed Keegan growing as expected. No mention of craniosynostosis occurred during the pregnancy.

Classifications of craniosynostosis

Divide each difficulty into as many parts as is
feasible and necessary to resolve it.
René Descartes

There are multiple classifications of CS. Generally, it is classified based on the cause of the condition, the number of sutures involved, and the sutures that fused prematurely, resulting in a specific head shape.

Classification by the cause

The most important classification of CS is based on cause: *nonsyndromic* versus *syndromic*.

- **Nonsyndromic CS:** CS that is not associated with a syndrome but is instead its own medical condition that has no known cause. Nonsyndromic CS accounts for 85 percent of cases of CS.[24]
- **Syndromic CS:** CS that is associated with a syndrome (a group of characteristics that consistently occur together).[25] Syndromic CS usually has a genetic cause and accounts for 15 percent of cases of CS.[24]

Classification by the number of sutures

- **Single suture CS:** The premature fusion of one suture. Most forms of nonsyndromic CS are single suture.[3]
- **Multisuture or multiple suture CS:** The premature fusion of more than one suture. Most forms of syndromic CS are multisuture[26] and the treatment is more complex than for single suture CS.

Classification by the suture that fused prematurely

- **Scaphocephaly:** The boat-shaped head typical of sagittal CS, which is caused by the premature fusion of the sagittal suture ("scapho" means boat).[27]
- **Trigonocephaly:** The triangular-shaped head typical of metopic CS, which is caused by the premature fusion of the metopic suture ("trigono" means triangle).[27]
- **Anterior plagiocephaly:** The skewed head shape in which the front of the head is flat on one side typical of unicoronal CS, which is caused by the premature fusion of one of the coronal sutures ("plagio" means oblique or slanted or at an angle; "uni" means one).[27]
- **Brachycephaly:** The short and wide head shape with a prominent forehead typical of bicoronal CS, caused by the premature fusion of both coronal sutures ("brachy" means short; "bi" means two).[27]
- **Posterior plagiocephaly:** The skewed head shape in which the back of the head is flat on one side typical of lambdoid CS, which is caused by the premature fusion of one of the lambdoid sutures.[27]

Figure 1.3.1 identifies various head shapes and the suture that fused prematurely to cause the head shape. The top image shows a skull without CS (normocephaly; "normo" means normal). The teal arrows indicate where the expanded compensatory growth will occur. The orange arrows indicate the area where growth is restricted due to the fused suture. The orange dotted lines indicate the fused suture.

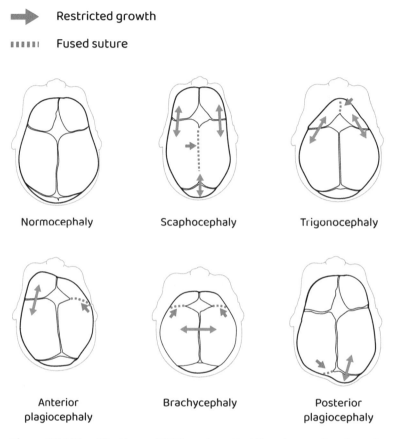

Figure 1.3.1 Classifications of CS by suture that fused prematurely and resulting head shape.

Table 1.3.1 summarizes key information about nonsyndromic CS and syndromic CS. Chapter 2 describes the types of nonsyndromic CS, and Chapter 3 describes the five most prevalent types of syndromic CS.

Table 1.3.1 Key information about nonsyndromic CS and syndromic CS

	NONSYNDROMIC CS	SYNDROMIC CS
Single suture	Frequent	Less frequent
Multisuture	Less frequent	Frequent
Progressive suture fusion after birth	Less frequent	Frequent
Head shape	Scaphocephaly: sagittal CS Trigonocephaly: metopic CS Anterior plagiocephaly: unicoronal CS Brachycephaly: bicoronal CS Posterior plagiocephaly: lambdoid CS	Depending on which sutures fuse, varying shapes can result.
Present at birth (congenital)	Yes	Yes
Prevalence	85%[24]	15%[24]

Figure 1.3.2 shows classification of CS beginning with the most important classification on the left side moving toward other classifications on the right. The size of the rectangles in the figure are generally proportional to prevalence.

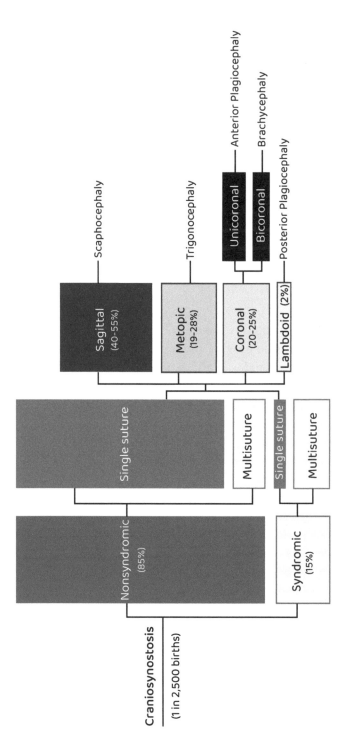

Figure 1.3.2 Classification of CS with associated prevalence.[3,5,7,20,24,28]

Prevalence, causes and risk factors, and symptoms

You may not control all the events that happen to you, but you can decide not to be reduced by them.

Maya Angelou

Prevalence

Prevalence is "the proportion of persons in a population who have a particular disease or attribute at a specified point in time or over a specified period of time."[29] Prevalence can vary geographically.

The worldwide prevalence of CS is 1 in every 2,500 live births, or about 0.04 percent of live births globally.[3] Globally, an estimated 85,000 children were born with CS in 2019.[30]

The prevalence of CS of any type is increasing. Three large studies over four decades up to the 2010s, from the US, Australia, and the Netherlands, reported an average annual increase of 2.5 to 12.5 percent.[31,32,33] The cause of the increase is unknown.

Causes and risk factors

The US Centers for Disease Control and Prevention (CDC) defines the term "cause" as "a factor (characteristic, behavior, event, etc.) that directly influences the occurrence of disease. A reduction of the factor in the population should lead to a reduction in the occurrence of disease."[34]

The term "risk factor" can be defined as "an aspect of personal behavior or lifestyle, an environmental exposure, or an inborn or inherited characteristic that is associated with an increased occurrence of disease or other health-related event or condition."[34]

Causes have a stronger relationship with a condition than risk factors do. For example, if someone were to fall and break their arm, the cause of the break would be the fall. However, the risk factors might include freezing temperatures, icy surfaces, unsteady gait, or poor lighting.

Syndromic CS is caused by a genetic variation, and genetic testing is typically recommended. Syndromic CS is covered in detail in Chapter 3.

The cause of *nonsyndromic* CS has not been identified, and research is ongoing. Genetic testing may also be recommended for individuals with nonsyndromic CS and the decision to pursue genetic testing should be discussed with the medical professional.

The practice around genetic testing may vary in different regions.

The risk factors for nonsyndromic CS can be divided into fixed (those that cannot be changed) and variable (those that can be changed).

Fixed risk factors for nonsyndromic CS include sex, race, ethnicity, and family history.

- Nonsyndromic CS is overall more common in males than females, but there are differences by sutures: sagittal CS and metopic CS are more common in males, and unicoronal CS is more common in females.[4,26]
- Higher rates of nonsyndromic CS have been found among White people than in other races and ethnicities.[35] Asian people with

nonsyndromic CS are more often impacted by multisuture CS than are White people with CS, but a lower incidence of sagittal CS exists in Asian people compared to White people.[36]

- Having a first-degree relative with nonsyndromic CS has been noted in 7 percent of individuals with nonsyndromic CS.[37]

Variable risk factors for nonsyndromic CS include parental age, maternal health, lifestyle characteristics, and perinatal factors.

- Advanced parental age, both maternal and paternal.[26,38]
- Maternal smoking, the use of certain medications, fertility treatments, gestational diabetes, and thyroid disease.[39,40,41,42,43,44,45]
- Low birth weight, preterm birth (before 37 weeks), or multiple birth pregnancies such as twins or triplets.[32,45]

Although having one or more risk factors may make it more likely that a child will be born with nonsyndromic CS, the risk factors are not the cause; the cause is still unknown. Parents who have questions about risk factors and/or how to prevent CS in future pregnancies should consult a medical professional.

When Keegan was first diagnosed, I looked for information online, primarily to find support from others who had already been on this journey, as well as to try to determine what may have caused our son to have craniosynostosis.

I compared this pregnancy to my prior pregnancy and did not come up with any major differences. I thought about the radiation I'm exposed to in the operating room where I work, from X-rays and such, but I always wear lead protection, so I didn't find that to be a likely cause. Looking on social media, I found many websites on craniosynostosis with multiple posts suggesting causes, but I soon learned that there is no known specific cause.

I am thankful for researchers and scientists who try to solve these mysteries for us. Until they do, we move forward with what has been placed in our laps and make the most of it for our sweet little ones.

Symptoms

Symptoms of CS (both nonsyndromic and syndromic) include:

- **An atypical head shape:** The hallmark of CS is an atypical head shape. This is very often the first sign that raises concerns for parents or medical professionals.[46,47]
- **Development of a ridge (a firm edge that can be seen and felt, where the sutures fused) on the skull:** A ridge does not always indicate CS; in Chapter 2, a particular ridge, known as the metopic ridge, is described. This can occur in typically developing infants, but this is not CS and does not require surgery.[48]
- **A persistently bulging fontanel.**[46,49]
- **Asymmetrical (uneven) facial characteristics:** Examples are uneven or droopy eyes, ears too far forward or back, and any other characteristic that makes the face appear uneven.[49] In some types of CS, the forehead may appear to be swept back and pulled away from the face. The infant in Figure 1.4.1 has facial asymmetry caused by CS. The left eye is lower than the right eye and the forehead is slightly broader on the left side.

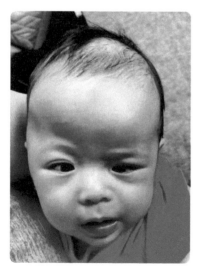

Figure 1.4.1 Infant with facial asymmetry caused by CS.

At Keegan's two-week well-child doctor appointment, the pediatrician greeted us with pleasantries, but I noticed he was quite focused on looking at Keegan. He stepped out saying he would be right back, and when he returned, he brought with him a figure chart. He felt Keegan's head and said there was a ridge on top from where the front soft spot area was supposed to be toward the back of his head. Keegan had a prominent forehead, and the back of his head was quite narrow in comparison. We knew Keegan's head had a different shape but did not feel that was out of the ordinary compared to other babies, as not many have perfectly circular heads after vaginal deliveries.

The pediatrician said he suspected craniosynostosis. My immediate thought was that he would just need to wear a helmet. But the pediatrician then told us that surgical correction is usually needed. He recommended following up for further evaluation in two weeks, at the one-month well-child doctor appointment. The news was not exactly something we wanted to hear, but we remained optimistic.

During the wait for the next appointment, I researched online the new words we had learned: "scaphocephaly" and "craniosynostosis." Each website I looked at reiterated the need for surgery and the possibility that craniosynostosis could be linked to different syndromes and developmental issues.

At the one-month visit, Keegan was happy, healthy, and gaining weight like crazy. However, his head shape was still concerning, and the pediatrician referred us to a craniofacial surgeon for evaluation. I broke down and cried, feeling this confirmed that our sweet little innocent, precious baby would need surgery. I'll never forget the sound of my tears falling on the paper liner on the exam table.

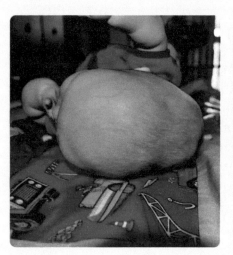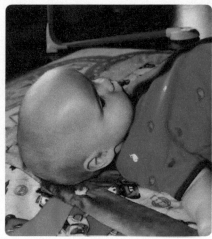

Keegan, with an atypical head shape (scaphocephaly) at age 10 weeks. Note the elongated head from front to back in the superior view (left) and the bulging forehead in the lateral view (right).

Diagnosis

Go as far as you can see,
and when you get there,
you will see farther.
Elbert Hubbard

A suspicion of CS is most often triggered by its most common symptom, an atypical head shape, usually noticed shortly after birth by parents or family members, or by medical professionals with experience in recognizing the condition. While it may be possible to diagnose some types of CS (particularly *syndromic* CS) before birth by using ultrasound, doing so is uncommon.[50,51,52] Research is continuing to determine if early screening could be beneficial in birth planning, prenatal counseling, early referral, and treatment without resulting in too much family anxiety or incorrect diagnoses.

Once CS is diagnosed or highly suspected, a referral to a pediatric craniofacial surgeon* in a hospital experienced in treating the condition is recommended. Skilled craniofacial surgeons can often recognize CS immediately upon seeing the child. These surgeons work in partnership with other medical professionals in what is commonly referred to as a craniofacial team. In many hospitals, a neurosurgeon† will also be involved in the diagnosis and management of CS.

The craniofacial team will gather information about the child and family, and conduct a physical exam to determine a diagnosis of CS (nonsyndromic and syndromic).

Child and family history

The child and family history includes:[49,53]

- History of the pregnancy and delivery
- Maternal medication use or maternal health issues during pregnancy
- Family history of CS (genetic testing possible)
- Airway (breathing) or feeding issues after birth (common in syndromic CS, rare in nonsyndromic CS)
- Head shape, size, or growth including growth that is too fast or too slow

Physical exam

The physical exam typically includes:

- **Facial symmetry or evenness of the facial features:** In infants with CS, restriction of growth of the skull bones can cause asymmetry in the eyes, forehead, and ears.

---

* A craniofacial surgeon is trained specifically in reconstructive surgery of the skull and facial bones. The term "pediatric" means a medical professional who specializes in the care and treatment of children.

† A neurosurgeon specializes in surgery on the nervous system, especially the brain and spinal cord.

- **Appearance and feel of the sutures:** In infants with CS, atypical ridging or flatness may form along the sutures and could indicate a premature fusion of the suture.[26]
- **Appearance and feel of the fontanels:** Examining the fontanels in infants can help detect certain conditions, including CS. However, fontanels in infants can also change due to illness or crying. Persistent changes in the fontanels, such as bulging or a sunken appearance, or an atypical shape of the fontanels may be cause for concern. (In metopic CS, for example, the anterior fontanel may become more triangular.)[22]
- **Eye movement:** Infants with CS may have atypical eye movement and blinking reflexes along with other conditions that may impact the eyes. A formal examination of the eyes by an ophthalmologist (an eye specialist) is recommended for all infants with CS.[54]
- **Head circumference and cranial index:** The head circumference is typically measured using a simple measuring tape. It is also measured prenatally using ultrasound to follow the growth of the fetus before birth. The growth charts of head circumference from birth to two years, published by the World Health Organization (WHO), are useful to follow the child's head circumference compared with children of the same age (Figures 1.5.2 and 1.5.3).[55] Note that head circumference is *not* an indicator of head shape, so it is not a reliable indicator of CS. The compensatory growth along the other open sutures in a child with CS may result in head circumference being within a typical range despite having an atypical head shape.[53] A better measure may be the cranial index, which is the maximum width of the skull divided by the maximum length of the skull, expressed as a percentage.[56]

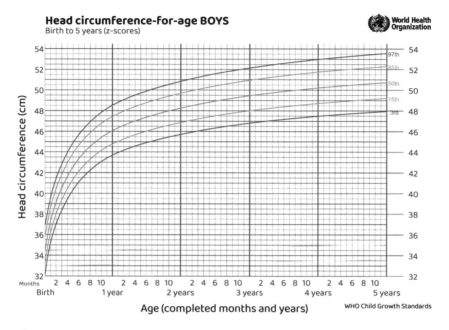

Figure 1.5.2 Head circumference growth chart for boys, birth to five years. Reproduced with kind permission from WHO.

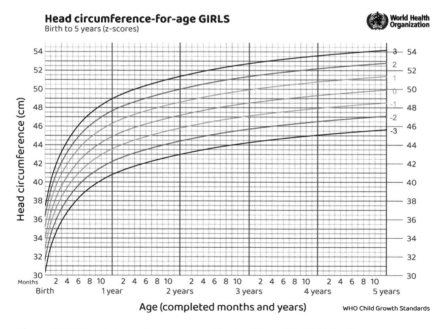

Figure 1.5.3 Head circumference growth chart for girls, birth to five years. Reproduced with kind permission from WHO.

- **Neurologic exam** (if determined necessary by the neurosurgeon): Neurologic exams typically include testing structures and functions that are controlled by the nervous system such as reflexes, movements, and sensations. If any concerns are noted, further investigation may be required.
- **Imaging:** If the craniofacial team strongly suspects CS, they will order any or a combination of a CT scan, X-ray, MRI scan, and ultrasound.
    - CT and X-ray use radiation to create the image. They are most useful in identifying hard, bony structures.
    - CT is the most used imaging tool for diagnosing CS, and advanced CT scans can create three-dimensional (3D) images* or models of the head. This is considered the most complete and accurate imaging to diagnose CS.[2] A benefit is that it can be done quickly and typically does not require sedation.†
    - MRI is particularly useful in visualizing soft structures, such as brain tissue, and may be ordered if there are concerns about brain structure and development. It is not as useful for viewing hard structures such as bone and fused sutures. An advantage of MRI is that it does not use radiation, but a disadvantage is that it often requires sedation.
    - Other imaging, such as ultrasound, which uses high-frequency sound waves to create images of internal structures, is ordered as necessary.[58]

> The waiting time between each appointment for Keegan wasn't easy— just not knowing what was to come. We told family and friends of the potential diagnosis but did not go into detail about treatments as we were not certain ourselves.
>
> We met with a craniofacial surgeon when Keegan was two months old. He was very kind at our appointment and gave us a rundown of craniosynostosis. He explained that it is premature fusion of the sutures of the skull, preventing the skull from growing and expanding the way

---

* A 3D image is a computer-generated graphic that shows three dimensions as opposed to two as in a typical photo. These images can be viewed or manipulated on the computer or printed as physical models on specialized printers.[57]

† Sedation is the administration of medications to produce a state of calm or sleep.

it should, which can cause pressure on the brain as it grows, resulting in an atypical head shape, compression on the brain, and even permanent brain damage. He also explained that craniosynostosis can be an isolated finding or may be associated with a syndrome. We were told there is a very small chance of craniosynostosis being passed down by family.

We confirmed there was no craniosynostosis on either side of our family. We had not used any fertility medications when conceiving, and I have no other medical conditions. The only thing I took during pregnancy was prenatal vitamins. Also, our craniofacial surgeon told us that Keegan's craniosynostosis didn't seem to have been caused by positioning in the pelvis or by any environmental factors. All this helped relieve some of my unspoken blame on myself.

The doctor recommended a CT scan for diagnostic purposes and surgical planning. About 20 minutes later, Keegan was lying on the CT table and buckled in with a strap over his forehead so his head wouldn't move. My husband and I put on lead aprons so we could stand by him, and I was able to keep my hand on him the whole time. Keegan did great and did not require any sedation. We then reviewed the results with the craniofacial surgeon who showed us the scan and confirmed fused suture lines. Keegan was diagnosed with nonsyndromic sagittal craniosynostosis, the most common form of craniosynostosis. He also had a partially fused lambdoid suture. We did not pursue genetic testing given his craniosynostosis was nonsyndromic.

After our appointment, we knew surgery was the next step. We began sharing our newfound information with family and friends. We told them that Keegan had a spot on his skull that fused together too soon so his head would not be able to grow properly, and that he would need surgery to make his skull more circular again. If he did not have surgery, it could eventually cause pressure on his brain or even permanent brain damage.

People began coming out of the woodwork when we mentioned craniosynostosis; suddenly someone knew someone else who had a child who had craniosynostosis, or someone knew of their own distant relative who was born with craniosynostosis. Even my manager at work said to me, "Have you never noticed my scar?" and pointed to the side of his head. That's when I learned he was born with craniosynostosis and had had surgery many years ago.

One of my friends told me her friend had a son who was born with craniosynostosis and that she and another mom started an organization where they would mail care packages to "cranio kids" (children diagnosed with craniosynostosis) before their surgeries. She gave me her information, and I was able to connect with her through social media. She was my first personal connection to the craniosynostosis world, another soul who had walked the same path I was currently walking.

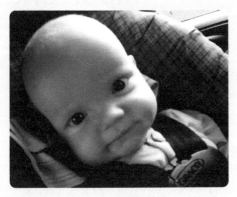

Keegan, before CS surgery.

Why treatment is important

In times of stress, the best thing we can do for each other
is to listen with our ears and our hearts and to be assured
that our questions are just as important as our answers.

Fred Rogers

The treatment for CS is surgical repair. Most often, particularly for nonsyndromic CS, a single surgery before a child is one year of age is all that is required to completely correct the condition. Others, however, may require additional surgeries (both for those with nonsyndromic and syndromic CS), and children with *syndromic* CS may require surgeries for other body systems. Surgical management of CS is described in Chapter 4.

There are several goals in the treatment of CS:

- **Preventing increased intracranial pressure and permanent brain damage:** Brain damage from increased intracranial pressure could result in cognitive impairment, seizures,* and life-threatening symptoms.[49,51] It is estimated that at least 15 percent of individuals with nonsyndromic CS and up to 60 percent with multisuture CS, as often occurs with syndromic CS, have increased intracranial pressure.[61,62] However, there is no way to predict which individuals with CS will develop this condition, which is why a surgical repair is always recommended. Surgical repair promotes normal brain growth by releasing the restriction in the cranial vault caused by the prematurely fused sutures.

- **Preventing papilledema:** Papilledema is the swelling of the optic nerve, which can result from increased intracranial pressure. Untreated, it can lead to permanent vision loss.[5,63]

- **Correcting head shape and facial symmetry:** Surgical repair can correct the head shape and face to improve appearance, which has been shown to positively affect emotional and social well-being.[5] It also allows for better fitting of protective headgear such as helmets for sports. Surgical repair is best done early, as it is more challenging and may not be possible after skull growth is complete.[64]

- **Protecting eyes and correcting eye abnormalities:**
  - **Supraorbital rim (brow bone) abnormality:** When the brow bone, which protects the eyes, is altered, the eyes are more susceptible to injury. Figure 1.6.1 shows an infant with metopic CS before and after corrective surgery.
  - **Hypertelorism/hypotelorism:** Hypertelorism refers to the spacing between the eyes being wider than typical; hypotelorism refers to the spacing being smaller than typical ("hyper" means over or overly; "hypo" means below or low).
  - **Proptosis (exorbitism):** This describes bulging eyes and may prevent the eyes from closing completely. This condition puts the cornea (the transparent layer at the front of the eye) at risk for injury and may lead to issues with vision.[54]
  - **Strabismus:** This is the misalignment of the eyes, sometimes appearing as crossed eyes. It may occur due to the change in space between the eyes, abnormal anatomy, or abnormal muscles that control eye movements.[54] If it is left uncorrected, it can

---

* A seizure is "a sudden, uncontrolled, abnormal burst of electrical activity in the brain that may cause changes in the level of consciousness, behavior, memory, or feelings."[59] Seizures may occur in individuals diagnosed with epilepsy, which is a neurological disorder in which brain activity becomes abnormal.[60] Seizures may also occur without epilepsy and may be caused by factors within the brain, such as increased intracranial pressure.

lead to what is commonly called lazy eye (amblyopia), where one eye becomes stronger and the other, the "lazy" one, has reduced vision.[65]

- **Managing a Chiari malformation:** A Chiari malformation is a condition in which brain tissue extends into the spinal canal instead of staying within the skull. It occurs because the base of the skull becomes too small and forces some of the brain tissue downwards.[66,67,68] If an infant has CS, having a neurosurgeon evaluate for a Chiari malformation is recommended. Some types of CS are more susceptible to a Chiari malformation, especially those that involve the lambdoid suture.[66]

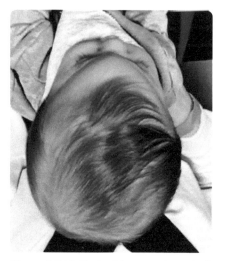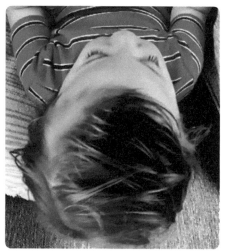

Figure 1.6.1 Infant with metopic CS before (left) and after corrective surgery (right). In the left image, the angle of the frontal bone is not rounded and the angle of the supraorbital rim is not protective of the eyes. In the right image, the frontal bone is rounded and eye protection by the supraorbital rim is restored.

Besides these surgical corrections, children with CS may require treatment for cognition-related issues. "Cognition" refers to the process of acquiring knowledge and understanding (e.g., memory, learning, and planning).[69] Specific issues related to cognition and behavior are described in both Chapter 2 (nonsyndromic) and Chapter 3 (syndromic).

Keegan was referred to an ophthalmologist to monitor eye pressure, and he was found to have very mild ptosis (drooping of the upper eyelid).* This has never required intervention. He continues with yearly eye appointments, including dilation of the eyes, which have never shown any problems.

---

* Some forms of syndromic CS are associated with a high risk of ptosis and are described further in Chapter 3. Ptosis can also occur without CS.

Best practice

Alone we can do so little; together we can do so much.

Helen Keller

Evidence-based medicine and shared decision-making

Evidence-based medicine (or evidence-based practice) is "the conscientious, explicit, and judicious use of current best evidence in making decisions about the care of individual patients".[70] It combines the best available external clinical evidence from research with the clinical expertise of the professional.[70] Family priorities and preferences are also considered.[71]

Since clinical expertise can vary, it is important to know that recommendations in this book may be different from those at different hospitals and treatment centers. Furthermore, treatment is not "one size fits all"; it must be customized. The best practice of managing CS is having a multidisciplinary craniofacial team skilled in providing CS medical care and engaging with the family in a shared decision-making model, a process in which the family is actively involved in making decisions about medical treatment and care. The key to shared decision-making is incorporating the principles of evidence-based medicine.[72]

Multidisciplinary team approach

The multidisciplinary team approach means the person is treated by medical professionals from a number of disciplines. They work as a team, but each stays within their professional boundaries. Such a team can provide information and resources to families to prepare for their child's surgery, recovery, rehabilitation, and coordinated care as their child grows. Some centers will have a key point person who will help coordinate care across the various teams.

Figure 1.7.1 lists the multidisciplinary team specialists, each with varying degrees of involvement in treatment and management of CS.

Multidisciplinary care is essential in the management of individuals with CS. Individuals with syndromic CS often require a larger team than those with nonsyndromic CS. The following lists individuals on the multidisciplinary CS team, particularly for syndromic CS. This list is not fully inclusive, and not all teams will have representation from the same disciplines. Team members may have different titles, and roles may vary in different countries.

- Advanced practice practitioner (nurse practitioner or physician assistant)
- Anesthesiologist and nurse anesthetist (administration of medication resulting in a sleep-like state needed for surgery)
- Audiologist (hearing)
- Child life specialist (child development and effective coping through play)
- Craniofacial surgeon
- Dentist
- Geneticist (family genetics)
- Neuropsychologist (brain and its functional relationship to cognition and behavior)
- Neurosurgeon

- Nurse
- Nutrition specialist
- Occupational and physical therapist (rehabilitative care focused on improving function in everyday activities and improving strength and functional mobility)
- Ophthalmologist (eyes)
- Orthodontist (teeth and jaw alignment)
- Otolaryngologist (ear, nose, throat, airway)
- Pediatrician and critical care providers
- Pulmonologist (lungs and airway)
- Psychologist
- Respiratory therapist
- Social worker
- Speech and language pathologist, or language therapist (communication and swallowing conditions)

Figure 1.7.1 Members of the multidisciplinary team[3,73]

In many hospitals, CS surgical repair is done by two surgeons working simultaneously: a craniofacial surgeon and a neurosurgeon. The craniofacial surgeon does the remodeling portion while the neurosurgeon ensures the protection of the brain and tissues. This approach allows each surgeon to focus on their area of expertise and requires the child to be under anesthesia for a shorter time.

Note: Families sometimes think that because a neurosurgeon is involved, the actual surgery is on the brain; CS surgery is only on the skull, not the brain.

At the appointment with the craniofacial surgeon, we also met with a pediatric neurosurgeon since the two would be performing Keegan's surgery together. We were told that the neurosurgeon's main purpose was to protect Keegan's brain during the surgery. Knowing that helped us feel more at ease with surgery, as one of our biggest concerns was the possibility of an injury to his brain. We were given a folder filled with information about the craniofacial services, a list of craniofacial resources, and a brochure about the upcoming surgery and support resources available. Knowing the specific roles of each person on the team and how they work together was reassuring for us.

Disparities in treatment of CS

Unfortunately, not all treatment of CS follows best practice in terms of timing of diagnosis and follow-up care: disparities exist for many reasons.

Both racial and ethnic disparities in treatment have been noted. In the US, for example, it has been found that White infants receive diagnosis and surgery weeks to months earlier than non-White and Hispanic infants.[74,75] Surgical timing was most delayed for Black infants, occurring approximately 10 months later compared to White infants.[75]

Another cause of disparity in the US is medical insurance. Those with public insurance have been found to be at risk of about a three-month delay in referral to a craniofacial surgeon compared to those with private insurance.[74,76] A delayed diagnosis can subsequently affect the time of surgery; those with public insurance were, on average, two months older at surgery compared to those with private insurance.[76]

Disparity also exists in low- and middle-income countries where there may be a lack of access to trained craniofacial surgeons, resulting in significant delays and gaps in care. This is of particular concern since the overall prevalence of CS is increasing.[30]

A discussion of strategies to address these disparities is outside the scope of this book.

Key points Chapter 1

- CS occurs when the sutures in an infant's skull fuse and cause the bones to join prematurely. This condition results in an atypical head shape. Surgical repair is the treatment for CS.
- CS occurs in 1 in every 2,500 births worldwide.
- Because the brain grows along with the skull, when the skull growth is disrupted, there is a risk of injury to the brain.
- CS is a condition that is present at birth, but it is not usually detected before birth.
- CS can be either nonsyndromic (accounting for 85 percent of CS cases and not associated with any other conditions) or syndromic (accounting for 15 percent of CS cases and associated with a condition, known as a syndrome).
- CS may involve a single suture fusing or multiple sutures fusing.
- No single cause of nonsyndromic CS has been identified.
- Syndromic CS is often linked to a genetic cause.
- A physical exam along with imaging studies such as CT, MRI, X-ray, or ultrasound are often done to confirm the diagnosis of CS.
- CS is best managed by a multidisciplinary craniofacial team in a hospital experienced in the treatment of CS, using a shared decision-making model.

Chapter 2

Nonsyndromic craniosynostosis

Introduction

Trials are the fire that refine us
Unknown

Nonsyndromic CS is CS that is present as an isolated condition, not as part of a syndrome. It accounts for 85 percent of cases.[24] Usually, it involves just one suture that fuses prematurely ("single suture CS").

This chapter covers the types of CS based on anatomical suture location. CS is often described by the name of the suture in front of either "synostosis" or "CS"; for example, "sagittal synostosis" or "sagittal CS." In most cases, surgery in the first year of life will effectively correct nonsyndromic CS, and those affected can expect a typical life.

Each type of CS based on anatomical suture location may occur in both nonsyndromic and syndromic CS. This chapter focuses on nonsyndromic CS.

USEFUL WEB RESOURCES

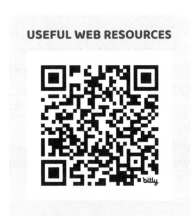

Sagittal CS

There isn't a way things should be.
There's just what happens, and what we do.

Terry Pratchett

Sagittal CS, or sagittal synostosis, occurs when the sagittal suture prematurely fuses. The sagittal suture is located where the two parietal bones meet, in the midline (middle) of the skull. This suture normally begins fusing at 22 years of age.[21] Sagittal CS is the most common type of CS, responsible for 40 to 55 percent of all cases.[5] It occurs more frequently in males than in females, at a 4:1 ratio.[3]

When the sagittal suture fuses early, the parietal bones cannot be pushed apart, and the skull cannot expand from side to side. Therefore, the skull expands front to back instead to accommodate brain growth. As shown in Figure 2.2.1, this causes scaphocephaly, or a boat-shaped, elongated head with a very prominent forehead and protruding occipital region (back of the head). In this infant skull, the metopic suture is fused as well, which is a typical finding in infants older than three months.

Sagittal CS

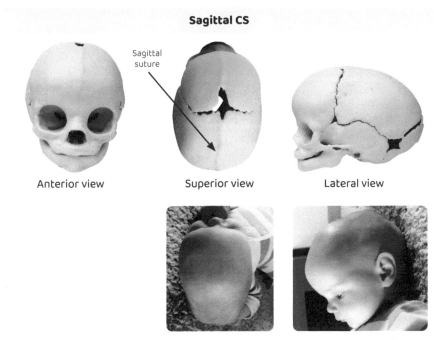

Sagittal
suture

Anterior view   Superior view   Lateral view

Figure 2.2.1 Anterior, superior, and lateral views of an infant skull showing fused sagittal suture (top). Superior and lateral photos of infant with sagittal CS at 10 weeks (bottom).

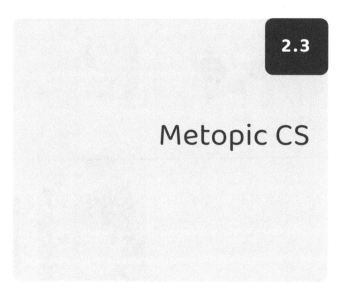

Metopic CS

Sunsets are proof that no matter what happens,
every day can end beautifully.

Kristen Butler

Metopic CS, or metopic synostosis, occurs when the metopic suture prematurely fuses. The metopic suture is in the front of the skull, where the two frontal bones meet. This suture normally fuses in infancy, at approximately 3 to 12 months of age.[5,7,20] Metopic CS is the second most common form of CS, accounting for 19 to 28 percent of all cases of CS.[7] It occurs more frequently in males than in females at a ratio of 3:1.[5]

When the metopic suture fuses early, the frontal bones cannot be pushed apart, so the skull expands toward the back and sides instead to accommodate brain growth. As shown in Figure 2.3.1, this causes trigonocephaly, or a triangle-shaped front of the head.

In Figure 2.3.1, the anterior view of the skull, the temples (the sides of the head toward the front) appear narrow, and there is a prominent ridge or bone along the forehead where the metopic suture has fused. Notice that the brow bones (supraorbital rims) are set back, and the eyes appear too close together, displaying a condition known as hypotelorism.

The superior view of the skull shows the triangle-shaped forehead, causing an atypical position of the brow bones. This positioning leaves the eyes susceptible to injury. The upper eyelids may also have skin folds that cover the inside corners of the eyes, a condition known as epicanthal folds.

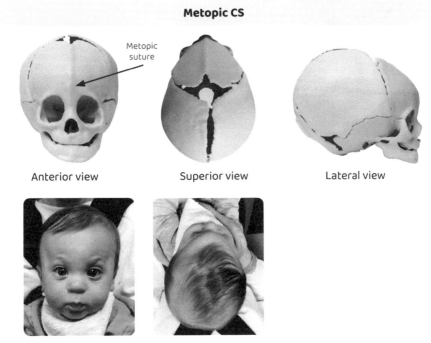

Figure 2.3.1 Anterior, superior, and lateral views of an infant skull showing metopic suture fused (top). Photos of infant with metopic CS (bottom).

"Metopic ridge" is a term used to define the ridge of bone that may be seen or felt when the metopic suture fuses in a typical infant *without* CS, as illustrated in Figure 2.3.2. This ridge usually resolves on its own around the time a child starts school, and it does not require surgery.

Differentiating metopic ridge from metopic CS can be a challenge. An important distinction between the two conditions is that metopic CS is present from birth while a metopic ridge typically develops after birth, at approximately three to four months of age. Therefore, the signs of metopic CS will appear earlier than those of a metopic ridge, and parents of infants with metopic CS may note an atypical head shape at birth.[48] A thorough physical exam by a craniofacial surgeon is recommended to differentiate the two.

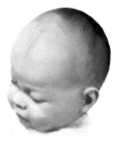

*A.D.A.M.

Figure 2.3.2 Infant with a metopic ridge. Reproduced with kind permission from A.D.A.M. Images.

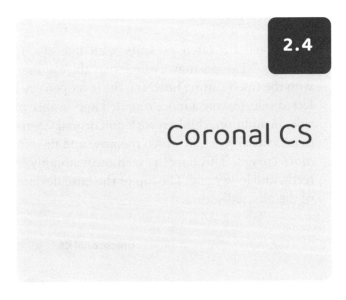

2.4

Coronal CS

Courage is not having the strength to go on;
it is going on when you don't have the strength.

Theodore Roosevelt

Coronal CS, or coronal synostosis, can involve either one or both coronal sutures, which are located toward the front half of the skull, where one frontal bone and one parietal bone meet. These sutures normally begin fusing at 24 years of age.[21] Coronal CS comprises 20 to 25 percent of all CS cases.[28]

Unicoronal

Unicoronal CS is the third most common form of CS accounting for 12 to 24 percent of all cases.[7] It is more common in females than males at a 3:2 ratio.[3]

When one coronal suture fuses early, the frontal and parietal bones on that side cannot be pushed apart, and the skull cannot expand front to back. This means the skull will expand on the other side of the head instead to accommodate brain growth. As shown in Figure 2.4.1, this causes a skewed head shape and a flat appearance of the forehead and temporal regions with the fused suture and bulging on the opposite side.

Unicoronal CS often presents with one eye appearing less open, or "droopy." Parents may assume that the eye that is less open is the side with the fused suture; however, the less open eye is typically on the unaffected side, leaving a more rounded appearance of the eye on the affected side. In addition, children with unicoronal CS may have what is referred to as a facial twist, in which the nose and the midline of the face appear more curved. This curve is seen most notably in the nose, chin, upper teeth, and lower jaw. The top of the nose deviates and points to the side of the affected suture.

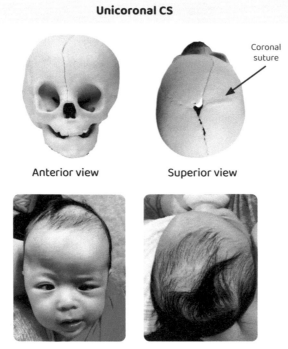

Unicoronal CS

Anterior view   Superior view

Figure 2.4.1 Anterior and superior views of an infant skull showing coronal suture fused (top). Photos of infant with unicoronal CS (bottom).

Bicoronal

Bicoronal CS accounts for only 3 percent of *nonsyndromic* cases, but it accounts for most *syndromic* CS cases,[7] which are described in Chapter 3. Bicoronal CS occurs equally in males and females.[77]

When both coronal sutures fuse early, the head cannot expand forward. As shown in Figure 2.4.2, this causes brachycephaly, meaning the skull is short in the front with a tall, flat forehead and wide from side to side.

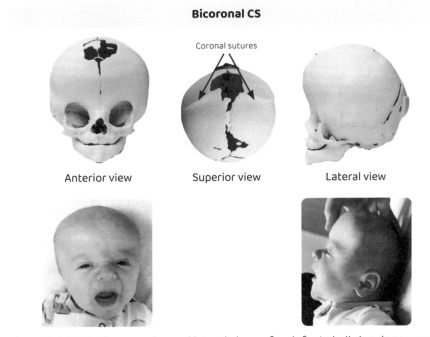

Bicoronal CS

Coronal sutures

Anterior view   Superior view   Lateral view

Figure 2.4.2 Anterior, superior, and lateral views of an infant skull showing coronal sutures fused (top). Photos of infant with bicoronal CS (bottom).

Lambdoid CS

Every child is a different kind of flower that
altogether make this world a beautiful garden.
Unknown

Lambdoid CS, or lambdoid synostosis, is the premature fusion of the lambdoid suture. Although the lambdoid suture can be divided into right and left lambdoid, it is more common to refer to any fusion along the lambdoid suture as lambdoid CS, instead of using "uni-"or "bi-," as is done with the coronal sutures. Most often, one side of the lambdoid suture will fuse prematurely.

Each lambdoid suture is located toward the back half of the skull, where one parietal bone and the occipital bone meet. This suture normally begins fusing at 26 years of age.[21] Lambdoid CS is the rarest form of CS, accounting for only 2 percent of all cases of CS.[7] It occurs equally in males and females,[78] and over 50 percent of individuals with lambdoid CS will have a Chiari malformation.[66]

When a lambdoid suture fuses early, the skull cannot push out to expand the back of the head on that side, so the bones on the opposite side push out instead. As shown in Figure 2.5.1, this causes a flat appearance on one side of the back of the head and a bulging appearance on the opposite side (posterior plagiocephaly). As well, infants with lambdoid CS may display a tilted skull.[79] The flattening of the head and the tilted skull base create asymmetry, especially in the posterior view.

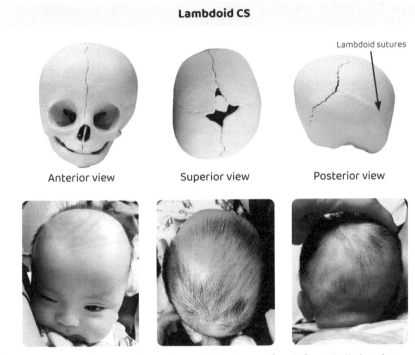

Figure 2.5.1 Anterior, superior, and posterior views of an infant skull showing lambdoid suture fused (top). Photos of infant with lambdoid CS (bottom).

Lambdoid CS versus deformational plagiocephaly

There is another condition that causes a similar head shape to lambdoid CS that is *not* a form of CS. It is called "deformational plagiocephaly," and it is not caused by prematurely fused sutures. Deformational plagiocephaly develops from external pressure on the skull bones, often caused by the infant being positioned on their back for long periods of time.

The two conditions are differentiated by comparing the head shapes to geometric shapes. Figure 2.5.2 shows both: on the left, viewed from above, the head shape of an infant with deformational plagiocephaly resembles a parallelogram, and on the right, the head shape of an infant with lambdoid CS resembles a trapezium (a four-sided figure with no parallel sides).[2] Notice that the sutures remain open in the infant with deformational plagiocephaly, while the lambdoid suture is fused in the infant with lambdoid CS.

Unlike CS, which requires surgery, deformational plagiocephaly is treated with repositioning, physical therapy, and helmet therapy. These treatments and this condition are described in detail in Chapter 5.

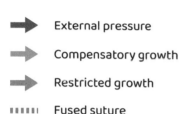

External pressure

Compensatory growth

Restricted growth

Fused suture

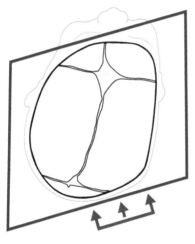

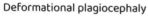

Deformational plagiocephaly

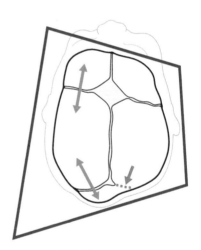

Lambdoid craniosynostosis

Figure 2.5.2 Comparison of head shape with deformational plagiocephaly (left) and lambdoid CS (right). In deformational plagiocephaly, the forces exert pressure from the outside of the skull (pink arrows). In lambdoid CS, the forces are from within the skull. Teal arrows show compensatory growth at the open sutures, and the orange arrow indicates the restricted growth at the fused suture (orange dotted line).

Cognition, behavior, speech, and language

Instruction does much, but encouragement everything.
Johann Wolfgang von Goethe

Cognition and behavior

Nonsyndromic CS may have an impact on cognition and behavior. Symptoms among children with surgically repaired single suture CS vary in presentation and severity, and studies show conflicting results.

- Those three years of age are below average on cognition outcomes.[80]
- At seven years of age, 58 percent show no learning difficulties.[81]
- At seven to nine years of age, they demonstrate lower IQ* and math scores compared to typical children.[81]
- In 6- to 18-year-olds IQ falls within the typical range.[84]

---

* Intellectual functioning is typically measured and expressed using standardized testing that includes an IQ (intelligence quotient). The average range of IQ scores in a typical population is 85–115. An IQ score of 70 or below indicates intellectual deficits.[82,83]

The impact appears to be suture-dependent and may be related to the timing of the surgical repair. Specifically:

- Children with sagittal CS have the mildest decreases in cognitive abilities.[81,84] Those with metopic CS have the most deficits, particularly in behavioral measures such as attention and impulsivity.[81,84,85] In absolute terms, cognitive and behavioral issues affect approximately one in three individuals with metopic CS.[85]
- Children having sagittal CS surgical repair at or before six months of age performed better on several academic learning measures and had fewer indicators for learning disabilities than those who had sagittal CS surgical repair after six months of age.[86]

Nonetheless, issues related to cognition and behavior may persist after surgical repair of CS, and since these issues may not be obvious in infants when surgeries are typically done, it's important that they are closely monitored as delays may not show up until the child starts school. Knowing the increased risk and watching for issues can ensure interventions begin early for the best outcomes.

To help identify and better understand specific concerns, children with nonsyndromic CS may be referred for neuropsychological evaluation. Neuropsychology is a specialty that focuses on understanding brain functioning as it relates to cognition and behavior.[87] A neuropsychological evaluation provides an individualized assessment of the skills and abilities that are linked to coordinated brain functions such as memory, cognition, perception, problem-solving, and verbal abilities. These may be initially indicated by developmental delays (delays in meeting milestones met at a certain age by the majority of typically developing children). Neuropsychological testing can also be valuable in identifying individual strengths and needs, helping to secure additional resources and interventions, and following progress over time or changes after interventions.

Screening for developmental delays is a routine part of well-child[*] visits in the US. These visits may be done in other countries, too, but may be known by other names.

Speech and language development

Children with surgically repaired nonsyndromic CS are at a higher risk of developing speech and language concerns compared to the general population.[88] A study of 101 children with surgically repaired nonsyndromic CS found that 56 percent had atypical speech and language ability, and the need for speech therapy was two to five times higher than in the general population.[89]

Hearing loss is also a risk; it occurs in 22 percent of children with nonsyndromic CS which is higher than in the general population.[90] Hearing loss can negatively impact speech and language development,[91] so speech and language therapy may be needed.

---

[*] In the US, well-child visits are regular appointments with medical professionals (typically as recommended by the American Academy of Pediatrics: three to five days after birth, then several times over the first 30 months, and then annually until adulthood). They often coincide with vaccination schedules and include growth and development tracking and monitoring.[11]

Key points Chapter 2

- Nonsyndromic CS is present as an isolated condition, is not part of a syndrome, and accounts for 85 percent of all CS cases.
- Nonsyndromic CS typically involves only one suture, and in the majority of individuals, a single surgery before the age of one will permanently correct the condition.
- Different types of nonsyndromic CS are sagittal CS, metopic CS, coronal CS (unicoronal or bicoronal), and lambdoid CS. Sagittal CS is the most prevalent form of nonsyndromic CS.
- Deformational plagiocephaly is a condition where an area of the head becomes flat due to external pressure, typically from positioning. It often results in a similar head shape seen with lambdoid CS and therefore needs to be distinguished from CS. It is not CS and does not require surgery.
- Issues related to cognition and behavior may be present in children with nonsyndromic CS and appear to be suture-dependent and may be related to the timing of the surgical repair.
- Neuropsychological testing or other screening may be recommended. This can help in securing additional resources and monitoring the outcomes of any recommended early interventions.
- Children with nonsyndromic CS are at an increased risk of speech and language concerns compared to the general population. Referrals to speech and language specialists may be needed.

Chapter 3

Syndromic craniosynostosis

Introduction

I am larger, better than I thought;
I did not know I held so much goodness.
All seems beautiful to me.
Whoever denies me, it shall not trouble me;
Whoever accepts me, he or she shall be blessed,
and shall bless me.
Walt Whitman

Syndromic CS is much rarer than nonsyndromic CS, making up only 15 percent of all cases of CS.[24]

A syndrome is a group of characteristics that consistently occur together and indicate a specific condition.[25] There is usually not a single test to diagnose a syndrome except for those that are caused by a specific genetic alteration. Most often, the diagnosis of a syndrome is made by evaluating the characteristics occurring together. Those diagnosed with a particular syndrome typically have several of the characteristics of that syndrome but not necessarily all of them.

There are almost 200 syndromes associated with CS.[24] This chapter describes the most prevalent syndromes and focuses mainly on the CS aspects of each. Note that some of these syndromes can be present in individuals who do *not* have CS.

It is important to recognize that this condition may cause anxiety and stress. Finding outlets in support groups, counseling, or other avenues may be beneficial. The Series Introduction includes information on coping for families raising a child with a disability. This, along with **Useful web resources,** provides information on the psychological aspects of this condition—both for the individual and their family.

The overall management of children with syndromes (of which CS is one part) is complex and beyond the scope of this book. Further information is included in **Useful web resources.**

USEFUL WEB RESOURCES

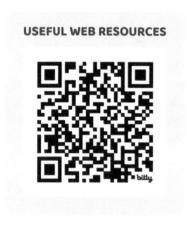

CS syndromes

It is surmounting difficulties that makes heroes

Louis Pasteur

The five most prevalent CS syndromes are Apert syndrome, Crouzon syndrome, Pfeiffer syndrome (types 1, 2, and 3), Muenke syndrome, and Saethre-Chotzen syndrome.

Apert syndrome

Apert syndrome is characterized by an atypical appearance of the skull and face along with atypically shaped hands and feet.[51] CS is almost always present in individuals with Apert syndrome.[92] Structural abnormalities in brain development may exist along with increased intracranial pressure.[93,94,95] As well, difficulty breathing and feeding at birth or shortly after, requiring intervention, may occur in children with Apert syndrome (see section 3.6 for further details). Webbed or conjoined (syndactyly) fingers and toes will require surgical repair, ideally within the first two years of life.[96,97] Problems with hands and feet that affect activities of daily living may persist even after surgery.

Crouzon syndrome

Crouzon syndrome is characterized by bulging eyes, a prominent forehead, an underdeveloped midface (hypoplasia), and a short upper lip.[51] Having a Chiari malformation and hearing loss is also common.[98] The condition sometimes presents without CS.[7] It can be mild with symptoms not always obvious, or it may be more severe, requiring interventions.[61] Because of this wide variation, sometimes adults have the syndrome but are not aware of it until they have genetic testing because their child is diagnosed with the syndrome.[61,99]

One variation is characterized by a distinct skin condition.[93] This is called Crouzon syndrome with acanthosis nigricans, and the incidence is higher in females than in males, but the rates of hearing loss and Chiari malformation are lower than in those with typical Crouzon syndrome.[100]

Pfeiffer syndrome

Pfeiffer syndrome is characterized by a high forehead and misshaped bones in the hands and feet, and dysfunction of internal organs, such as the intestines and stomach.[51,93] CS is almost always present in individuals with Pfeiffer syndrome.[101] As with Apert syndrome, Pfeiffer syndrome may present breathing and feeding challenges for the child at birth or shortly after, which may require intervention.

Pfeiffer syndrome is divided into three types: type 1 (61 percent of cases), type 2 (25 percent of cases), and type 3 (14 percent of cases).[102]

- Type 1 is the least severe with milder forms of CS and midface hypoplasia.
- Type 2 is characterized by a unique head shape termed "cloverleaf skull" because its shape resembles a three-leaf clover.
- Types 2 and 3 have more severe forms of CS, midface hypoplasia, airway obstructions, eye problems, and significant cognitive delays.[93,103]
- Types 2 and 3 frequently need early surgical intervention because of the pressure on the brain, and life expectancy may be impacted.[98]
- Other abnormalities that impact brain structure and function may occur in all types but particularly in types 2 and 3.[104]

Muenke syndrome

Muenke syndrome is characterized by an atypical appearance of the skull due to CS together with other characteristics such as wide-set eyes and flattened cheekbones. Unlike some other forms of syndromic CS, it does not typically involve hand or foot abnormalities or severe midface hypoplasia. Of those who have Muenke syndrome, 20 percent do *not* have CS.[93] As with Crouzon syndrome, an adult may not be aware they have the syndrome until genetic testing is done on their child.

Saethre-Chotzen syndrome

Saethre-Chotzen syndrome is characterized by an atypical appearance of the skull, face, hands, and feet. CS is often present, but in some it may be very mild or not present at all.[105] Again, due to varying severity, an adult may not be aware they have the syndrome until genetic testing is done on their child.[106]

Prevalence and genetics

Experience is not what happens to you;
it is what you do with what happens to you.
Aldous Huxley

Prevalence of syndromic CS

The prevalence of syndromic CS varies from 1 in 10,000 to 1 in 200,000, and the range of each is presented in Table 3.3.1. In each of the five syndromes, males and females are equally affected, although the presentation and severity of CS may vary by sex within a syndrome.[61,103,107,108,109,110]

Genetics of syndromic CS

Genetics is a branch of science that studies how physical or behavioral characteristics result from an organism's genes—the units of heredity—and how these characteristics are transferred from parents to children.[111] The building blocks of our genes are contained in our DNA.[111]

Figure 3.3.1 presents a simple graphic explanation of heredity. It shows one parent (the dad) who has a condition associated with a gene with a mutation—a "nonworking" gene, designated with an "x." Because just one of the parents has this gene, the odds of the child inheriting it, and therefore having the condition, are 50 percent. This is shown in the figure, with two of the four children having the condition. But it could have turned out that all the children inherited the gene—or none of them. Each child, individually, that this couple has will have the same 50 percent chance of inheriting the condition.

This inheritance pattern is termed autosomal dominant inheritance pattern, which most types of syndromic CS follow. That means that if a person has just one copy of the nonworking gene, they will have the condition.

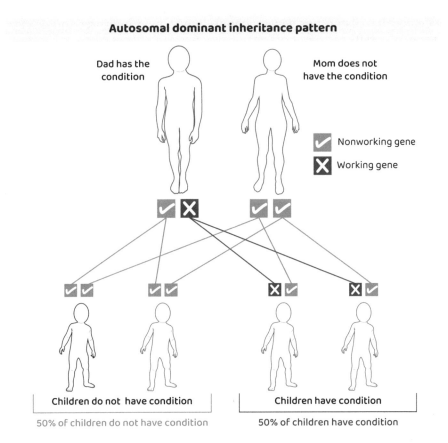

Figure 3.3.1 Autosomal dominant inheritance pattern from parents to children. Adapted with kind permission from Genetic Support Foundation.

Syndromic CS may also occur because of a *de novo* mutation to a gene, which is an alteration in a gene that appears for the first time in a child but is not present in either parent.[97] Advanced paternal age is one factor that has been positively associated with an increase in the occurrence of *de novo* mutations in syndromic CS.[93]

When syndromic CS is suspected, genetic testing is often recommended. This involves examining the DNA from blood, body fluids (usually saliva), or tissue samples to look for changes (mutations) in genes that may cause or increase the risk of a certain condition. Genetic testing can be helpful for medical treatment and future family planning.

Medical professionals can help you decide whether to have genetic testing for your child. If genetic testing is pursued, it is important to find a center that also offers genetic counseling to help interpret and discuss the results.[24,112]

Several gene mutations associated with syndromic CS have been discovered. These include *FGFR1*, *FGFR2*, *FGFR3*, and *TWIST1*.[113] The prevalence, genetic inheritance patterns, and common gene mutations of the syndromes are summarized in Table 3.3.1.

Table 3.3.1 Prevalence, inheritance patterns, and gene mutations by syndrome

SYNDROME	PREVALENCE (NUMBER OF CASES/ NUMBER OF BIRTHS)	GENETICS
Apert	1 in 65,000 to 200,000[107]	*Inheritance pattern:* • Rarely autosomal dominant [96] • Most *de novo*, and the affected gene comes solely from the father[114,115] *Gene:* *FGFR2* (over 98% of cases)[114]
Crouzon	1 in 25,000 to 60,000[116]	*Inheritance pattern:* • Most autosomal dominant[110] • Occasionally *de novo*[110] *Genes:* *FGFR2*[117] *FGFR3* (Crouzon with acanthosis nigricans)[117]
Pfeiffer	1 in 100,000[103]	*Inheritance pattern:* • Autosomal dominant or *de novo* in type 1[110] • Almost exclusively *de novo* in types 2 and 3[118] *Genes:* *FGFR1*[99] type 1 *FGFR2*[99] type 1, 2, 3
Muenke	1 in 10,000 to 30,000[93]	*Inheritance pattern:* • Most autosomal dominant[110] • Occasionally *de novo*[110] *Gene:* *FGFR3*[62]
Saethre-Chotzen	1 in 25,000 to 50,000[119]	*Inheritance pattern:* • Most autosomal dominant[120] • Occasionally *de novo*[120] *Gene:* *TWIST1*[114]

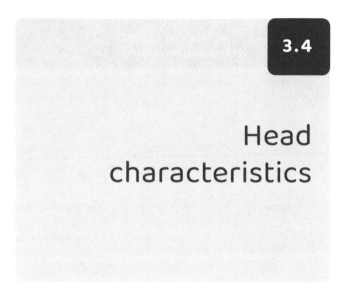

Head characteristics

> We were built differently. Locate your uniqueness.
>
> **Sunday Adelaja**

This section addresses:

- Suture involvement and head shape
- Increased intracranial pressure
- Hydrocephalus and ventriculomegaly
- Chiari malformation
- Facial structure

Suture involvement and head shape

Syndromic CS often involves premature fusion of multiple sutures, which might fuse progressively as the child grows. Fusion typically occurs within the first year but may also occur later.

Premature fusion of the coronal sutures (either unicoronal or bicoronal) is the most common suture involvement in individuals with syndromic

CS,[121] resulting in brachycephaly or turribrachycephaly.[122] Brachycephaly is a head shape that is short in the front with a tall, flat forehead and wide from side to side. Turribrachycephaly ("turris" means tower) is a towering, cone-shaped head with a flat, prominent, elongated forehead and wide side to side along with occipital flattening. A head shape known as a cloverleaf skull may also occur. This is a head shape that appears to have three sections and resembles a three-leaf clover, bulging at both sides and the forehead.[123]

Syndromic CS can involve any of the other major sutures as well as minor sutures and often involves the fusion of more than three cranial sutures, termed "pansynostosis."

Tables 3.4.1 to 3.4.5 summarize suture involvement and the most prevalent head shape across the five syndromes.

Increased intracranial pressure

The premature fusion of the sutures in CS may cause increased intracranial pressure; that is, pressure above the typical level within the skull. The risk of this occurring increases with the *number* of prematurely fused sutures and occurs more often in multisuture CS, as is often found in syndromic CS.[124] Increased intracranial pressure over a long period of time can lead to brain damage. It can also cause swelling of the optic nerve (papilledema), which if left untreated can result in permanent vision loss.[54]

When intracranial pressure is present at birth or shortly after, CS surgery will be done earlier than typical timelines.[61] Children with syndromic CS may also develop increased intracranial pressure *after* CS surgery due to either sutures that re-fuse or other factors.[51] Some types of syndromic CS are more likely to be associated with increased intracranial pressure that develops or redevelops after surgery.

The prevalence of increased intracranial pressure is syndrome dependent. Studies have shown that:

- Eighty-three percent of individuals with **Apert syndrome** experience increased intracranial pressure[93] with 50 percent affected in the first year of life. Increased intracranial pressure is still present in 35 percent of individuals with Apert syndrome after initial CS surgical repair.[61]

- Sixty-one percent of individuals with **Crouzon syndrome** experience increased intracranial pressure before surgical repair.[93]
- Eighty percent of individuals with **Pfeiffer syndrome** experience increased intracranial pressure, which often requires early surgical intervention to treat.[93]
- Twenty-six percent of individuals with **Muenke syndrome** experience increased intracranial pressure.[125] Higher rates of reoperations to address increased intracranial pressure which persists after initial CS surgical repair have been shown in individuals with Muenke syndrome.[61]
- More than 40 percent of individuals with **Saethre-Chotzen syndrome** experience increased intracranial pressure even after initial CS surgical repair.[61]

Hydrocephalus and ventriculomegaly

Hydrocephalus is the buildup of cerebrospinal fluid in cavities (ventricles) in the brain. This excess fluid causes increased intracranial pressure. The condition occurs in 12 to 15 percent of individuals with syndromic CS.[51] A condition known as ventriculomegaly, in which the ventricles in the brain are enlarged, may also occur.

The prevalence of hydrocephalus and ventriculomegaly is syndrome dependent. Studies have shown that:

- Over 10 percent of individuals with **Apert syndrome** have hydrocephalus and over 50 percent have ventriculomegaly.[95,126]
- Over 40 percent of individuals with **Crouzon syndrome** have hydrocephalus.[126]
- Sixty-eight percent of individuals with **Pfeiffer syndrome** have hydrocephalus.[61]
- Individuals with **Muenke syndrome** or **Saethre-Chotzen syndrome** rarely experience hydrocephalus[127,128] but ventriculomegaly occurs in 8 to 17 percent.[128]

Hydrocephalus is treated by placing a shunt in the ventricles to drain the excess fluid to reduce the intracranial pressure. A neurosurgeon performs this surgery, which may need to be done before other CS surgical repair in some infants with syndromic CS.

Figure 3.4.1 shows a child with a shunt placed for hydrocephalus. The shunt tubing (the catheter) drains the cerebrospinal fluid from the ventricles and transports it to a reservoir where it is stored and then pumped to the peritoneal cavity (a space within the abdominal area not occupied by the abdominal organs). There, the fluid is absorbed by the body.

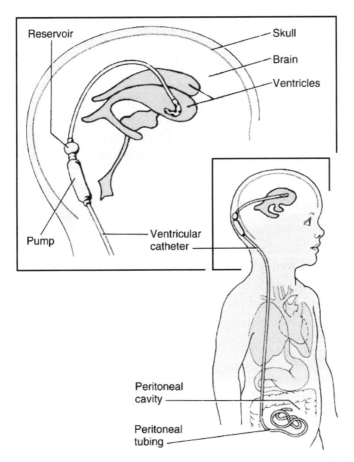

Figure 3.4.1 View of shunt placement in child with hydrocephalus. Reproduced with kind permission from Nurse Key (2016). Neurologic and Sensory Disorders [Online] Available: Neurologic and Sensory Disorders | Nurse Key.

Chiari malformation

A Chiari malformation may occur in children with multisuture or syndromic CS.[66] It can also be associated with hydrocephalus and often requires surgery to correct.[66] The prevalence rate depends on the syndrome and which sutures fuse early. When the lambdoid suture fuses early, the likelihood of developing a Chiari malformation increases.[66]

The prevalence of a Chiari malformation is syndrome dependent. Studies have shown that:

- Twenty-two percent of individuals with **Apert syndrome** experience a Chiari malformation.[95]
- Seventy-two percent of Individuals with **Crouzon syndrome** experience a Chiari malformation.[99]
- Over 80 percent of individuals with **Pfeiffer syndrome** (of all three types) develop a Chiari malformation.[102] One hundred percent of individuals with Pfeiffer types 2 and 3 develop a Chiari malformation.[102]
- Four percent of individuals with **Muenke syndrome** or **Saethre-Chotzen syndrome** experience a Chiari malformation.[129,130]

Facial structure

A child with syndromic CS may have an underdeveloped middle of the face (midface hypoplasia), which causes the upper jaw (maxillary hypoplasia), cheekbones, and eye sockets to appear sunken. Syndromic CS may also be accompanied by conditions that impact the eyes, ears, nose, and mouth.

Figures 3.4.2 to 3.4.6 depict individuals with each of the five syndromes. Tables 3.4.1 to 3.4.5 show the facial characteristics for each of the five syndromes, although these are not exhaustive lists. The following is a list of eye, ears, nose, and mouth terms and their definitions used in the tables.

Eyes, ears, nose, mouth:

- **Cleft palate:** A split or opened roof of the mouth.
- **Dental crowding:** Overlapping or misaligned teeth.
- **Deviated septum:** The wall between two nostrils in the nose; when deviated, it shifts to one side.
- **Ectopic teeth:** Teeth outside the typical position.
- **Eruption of teeth:** The process in which the teeth push through the gums into the mouth.
- **High-arched palate:** Narrow, tall roof of the mouth.
- **Helical folds:** The folds of the external ear.
- **Hypertelorism:** Spacing between the eyes that is wider than typical.
- **Nasal root deviation:** Atypical alignment of the top of the nose where the nasal bones meet the frontal bones; the nose deviates toward the fused suture.[125]
- **Nasolacrimal duct stenosis:** Blocked or narrowed (stenosis) tear duct; a condition of the eyes that causes decreased tear production and may lead to increased eye infections.
- **Natal teeth:** Teeth that are present at birth.
- **Otitis media:** Inflammation of the middle ear.
- **Otitis media with effusion:** A collection of fluid in the middle ear in the absence of an ear infection.[51]
- **Proptosis (also known as exorbitism or exophthalmos):** Bulging appearance of the eyes.
- **Ptosis:** Drooping of the upper eyelids.
- **Sensorineural hearing loss:** Hearing loss that occurs due to damage to the inner ear, impacting low-frequency (deep, low-pitched) sounds the most.[131] Soft sounds can be hard to hear, while loud sounds may be muffled.[132]
- **Strabismus:** Atypical alignment of the eyes, often appearing as crossed eyes.

Table 3.4.1 Apert syndrome: Suture involvement, head shape, and facial characteristics

SUTURES THAT MAY FUSE EARLY	MOST PREVALENT HEAD SHAPE	FACIAL STRUCTURE	EYES	EARS	NOSE	MOUTH
Bicoronal[133] **Sagittal**[92]	Turribrachycephaly[133]	Midface hypoplasia[61,134]	Hypertelorism[134] Strabismus[93]	Hearing loss occurs in 80%[131]	Small, beak-like nose[93]	High-arched, narrow palate[133]
Lambdoid[133] **Minor sutures**[94]		Maxillary hypoplasia[61,134]	Proptosis[134] Shallow eye orbits[93]	Low-set, large ears, constricted external ear canal[110,131] Recurrent otitis media[131]	Short nose with low, depressed bridge and rounded tip[110] Deviated septum[135]	Cleft palate[114] Delayed eruption of teeth, ectopic teeth, dental crowding,[133,136] frequent cavities from challenges with oral care due to hand syndactyly[135]

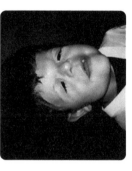
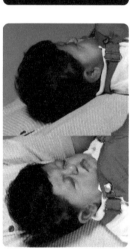
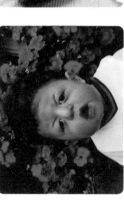

Figure 3.4.2 Child with Apert syndrome.

Table 3.4.2 Crouzon syndrome: Suture involvement, head shape, and facial characteristics

SUTURES THAT MAY FUSE EARLY	MOST PREVALENT HEAD SHAPE	FACIAL STRUCTURE	EYES	EARS	NOSE	MOUTH
Bicoronal[108]	Brachycephaly or turribrachycephaly[108,117]	Midface hypoplasia[134]	Hypertelorism[137]	Hearing loss occurs in 74%[131]	Short, upturned, beak-like nose[108]	High-arched palate[137]
Sagittal[117]		Maxillary hypoplasia[137]	Strabismus[137]	Low-set, wide ears[121,131]		Cleft palate[116]
Metopic[117]			Proptosis[134,137]	Recurrent otitis media with effusion[131]		Delayed eruption of teeth and dental crowding[110,138]
Minor sutures in jaw and eye areas[117]			Shallow eye orbits[110]			
May present without CS[7]						

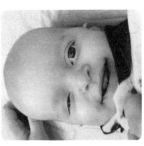
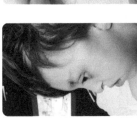
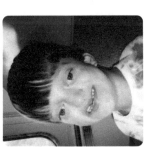
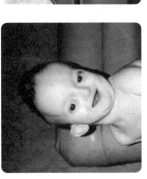
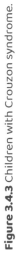

Figure 3.4.3 Children with Crouzon syndrome.

Table 3.4.3 Pfeiffer syndrome: Suture involvement, head shape, and facial characteristics

SUTURES THAT MAY FUSE EARLY	MOST PREVALENT HEAD SHAPE	FACIAL STRUCTURE	EYES	EARS	NOSE	MOUTH
Bicoronal[98]	Brachycephaly or Turribrachycephaly in types 1 and 3[61,103]	Midface hypoplasia[61]	Hypertelorism[110]	Hearing loss occurs in 92%[131]	Small, beak-like nose[103]	High-arched palate[140]
Lambdoid[103]		Maxillary hypoplasia[103]	Strabismus[110]	Recurrent otitis media with effusion[131]	Broad nasal bridge[140]	Cleft palate[103]
Sagittal[121]	Cloverleaf skull in type 2[134]		Proptosis[134]			Natal teeth and other dental problems[103]
Pansynostosis[139]			Shallow eye orbits[134]			
			Ptosis[140]			

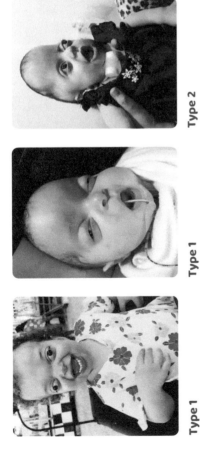

Type 1

Type 1

Type 2

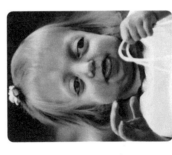

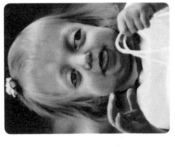

Type 3

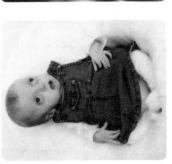

Type 3

Figure 3.4.4 Children with Pfeiffer syndrome: type 1 (top left and middle), type 2 (top right), type 3 (bottom).

Table 3.4.4 Muenke syndrome: Suture involvement, head shape, and Facial characteristics

SUTURES THAT MAY FUSE EARLY	MOST PREVALENT HEAD SHAPE	FACIAL STRUCTURE	EYES	EARS	NOSE	MOUTH
Unicoronal or Bicoronal[7]	Brachycephaly, turribrachycephaly, or cloverleaf skull[109]	Midface hypoplasia is not common, but if present, generally mild[61,110]	Hypertelorism[93]	Hearing loss is present in 61%; 79% is sensorineural hearing loss[131]	Short nose or depressed nasal bridge[109]	High-arched palate[5]
Lambdoid[109]			Strabismus[93]		Nasal root deviation[109]	Delayed eruption of teeth[138]
Sagittal[109]			Ptosis[110]	Low-set ears[131]		
Metopic[109]				Otitis media with effusion[131]		
Minor sutures[109]						

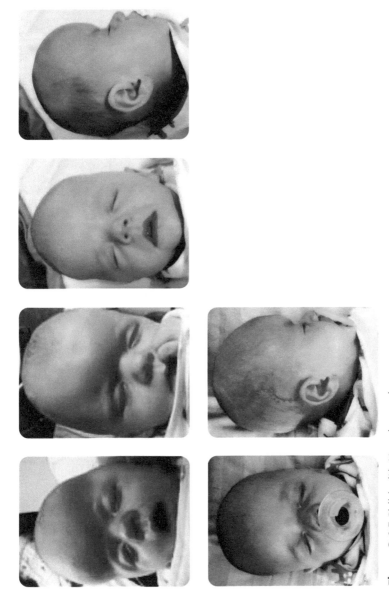

Figure 3.4.5 Child with Muenke syndrome.

Table 3.4.5 Saethre–Chotzen syndrome: Suture involvement, head shape, and facial characteristics

SUTURES THAT MAY FUSE EARLY	MOST PREVALENT HEAD SHAPE	FACIAL STRUCTURE	EYES	EARS	NOSE	MOUTH
Unicoronal or Bicoronal[119]	Brachycephaly[141] or turribrachycephaly	Midface hypoplasia is not common, but if present, generally mild[61,93]	Hypertelorism[93]	Hearing loss[141]	Flattened nose with a low, depressed bridge[120]	High-arched palate[120] Delayed eruption of teeth and other dental problems[119,138]
Metopic[106]			Strabismus[142]	Low-set, small ears[120]		
Lambdoid[106]		Maxillary hypoplasia[106]	Ptosis[7] Shallow eye orbits[93]	Prominent ear helical folds (the external ear folds)[120]		
			Nasolacrimal duct stenosis[120]	Recurrent otitis media with effusion[143]		

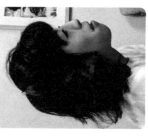
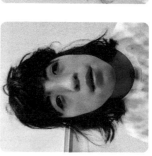

Figure 3.4.6 Individual with Saethre–Chotzen syndrome.

Additional characteristics

Be yourself; everyone else is already taken.
Oscar Wilde

Many syndromic CS variations result in atypical characteristics in the hands and feet and other skeletal areas, along with various co-occurring conditions. The most prevalent characteristics are described in Tables 3.5.1 to 3.5.5, although these are not exhaustive lists. Below is a list of terms and definitions used in the tables.

Hands and feet:

- **Brachydactyly:** Shorter than typical fingers and toes.
- **Broadening**: To become larger in distance from side to side; widen.
- **Clinodactyly:** A condition in which fingers are bent or curved.
- **Partial syndactyly:** The partial union of two or more fingers or toes, also called "webbing"; adjacent digits that are not fully conjoined or joined only by skin instead of bones.
- **Syndactyly:** The union of two or more fingers or toes, also called "webbing"; may include bony *fusion* of adjacent digits.

Other skeletal areas:

- **Ankylosis:** Immobility and fusion of a joint; leads to stiffness and rigidity in the joint.
- **Symphalangism:** Stiffness of the joints due to ankylosis.
- **Synostosis:** Fusion of two or more bones.
- **Vertebrae:** The bones that form the spine.

Other:

- **Aortic coarctation:** Narrowing of the main vessel in the heart.[144]
- **Epilepsy:** A neurological disorder in which brain activity becomes abnormal, causing seizures (see below) or periods of unusual behavior, sensations, and sometimes loss of awareness.[60]
- **Gastroesophageal reflux:** A condition where the liquid contents of the stomach go back up into the esophagus instead of staying in the stomach and moving into the intestines. Also called "acid reflux."
- **Gastrointestinal:** Relating to the stomach and intestines.
- **Patent ductus arteriosus:** An unclosed hole in the main vessel in the heart, present at birth.[145]
- **Seizure:** "A sudden, uncontrolled, abnormal burst of electrical activity in the brain that may cause changes in the level of consciousness, behavior, memory, or feelings."[59] Seizures may occur in individuals diagnosed with epilepsy (see above). Seizures may also occur without epilepsy and may be caused by factors within the brain, such as increased intracranial pressure.

Table 3.5.1 Apert syndrome: Additional characteristics

HANDS AND FEET	OTHER SKELETAL AREAS	OTHER
Syndactyly occurs symmetrically in both hands and feet[95]	Symphalangism in wrists, ankles, elbows, and other joints[93]	Acne present in 70% during adolescence[99]
Brachydactyly[133]	Synostosis of forearm and upper arm bone (radius and humerus)[98]	Heart conditions present in about 25%[95]
Clinodactyly[133]		Excessive sweating[98]
	Short stature[93]	Gastrointestinal anomalies and gastroesophageal reflux[92,95]
	Fusion of cervical (neck) vertebrae[95]	
	Spinal anomalies[93]	

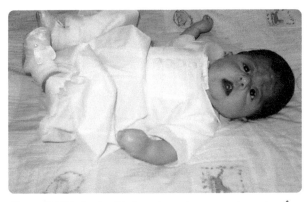

Figure 3.5.1 Infant with Apert syndrome and rosebud* syndactyly.

---

* The shape of the hand in an individual with Apert syndrome is described as either a spade, mitten, or rosebud.[121]

Table 3.5.2 Crouzon syndrome: Additional characteristics

HANDS AND FEET	OTHER SKELETAL AREAS	OTHER
Typically, not affected[108]	Fusion of cervical vertebrae[93] Elbow ankylosis[7]	Patent ductus arteriosus or aortic coarctation[121]

Table 3.5.3 Pfeiffer syndrome: Additional characteristics

HANDS AND FEET	OTHER SKELETAL AREAS	OTHER
Partial syndactyly[98] Brachydactyly[140]	Spinal anomalies[93] Fusion of spinal vertebrae[93,104]	Kidney and gastrointestinal conditions may be present in types 2 and 3[103]
Broadening and deviating of the thumbs and/or big toes[98] Clinodactyly of the fifth finger[140]	Elbow ankylosis and synostosis with types 2 and 3[98]	Seizures or epilepsy in types 2 or 3[104]

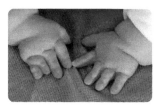

Figure 3.5.2 Reproduced with kind permission from Dr. Leslie G. Biesecker. Elements of morphology: Standard terminology for the hands and feet [Online]. Available at: https://onlinelibrary.wiley.com/doi/10.1002/ajmg.a.32596.

Table 3.5.4 Muenke syndrome: Additional characteristics

HANDS AND FEET	OTHER SKELETAL AREAS	OTHER
Brachydactyly[93] Fusion of the bones in the wrists and ankles[142] Broad thumbs[131]	Typically, not affected[146]	Seizures or epilepsy[109]

Table 3.5.5 Saethre-Chotzen syndrome: Additional characteristics

HANDS AND FEET	OTHER SKELETAL AREAS	OTHER
Partial syndactyly in second and third fingers[105] Brachydactyly[7] Broadening of the big toes[7] Clinodactyly of the fifth finger[147]	Fusion of vertebrae in the neck[143] Synostosis of forearms[105] Short stature[106]	Heart conditions[121] A low frontal hairline[120]

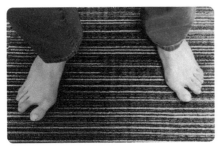 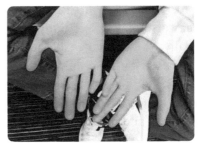

Figure 3.5.3 Broadening of the big toes (left) and clinodactyly (right) in an individual with Saethre-Chotzen syndrome.

Airway, feeding, and eye closure

We may encounter many defeats,
but we must not be defeated.
Maya Angelou

As described above, syndromic CS involves more than just the premature fusion of cranial sutures and CS. Children born with syndromic CS may also have issues with breathing, feeding, and closing their eyes. Typically, these need to be addressed before surgical management of CS. This section describes these issues and their management.

Keep in mind that not all children with syndromic CS will experience these issues, and the severity will vary. The craniofacial team will address them as they arise.

Airway

Children born with syndromic CS will often require an airway evaluation by an otolaryngologist (a doctor specializing in the care of the ears, nose, and throat, often referred to as ENT).[148] This may be done at birth and again before any CS surgical corrections.

Frequently, children with syndromic CS have a tilted skull base, which can affect breathing control.[148] Airway issues can also result from facial structure differences, such as midface hypoplasia, or maxillary hypoplasia, both common in syndromic CS, and which result in less space in the nose, mouth, and throat.[103,149] Figure 3.6.1 depicts the typical airway space in an individual without CS compared to one with syndromic CS, specifically Apert syndrome.

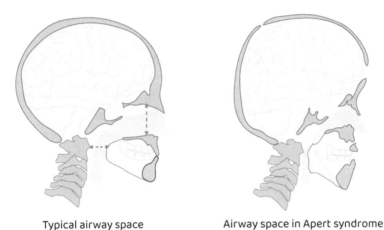

Typical airway space   Airway space in Apert syndrome

Figure 3.6.1 View of airway space in a typical individual (left) and in an individual with Apert syndrome (right). Adapted with kind permission from John Persing, MD. Original image by Xioana Lu, MD.

The following complications can arise from reduced airway space. Once surgical correction occurs and the child grows, some of these complications may resolve.

- **Obstructive sleep apnea:** This is a condition in which an individual frequently stops breathing during sleep. These interruptions in breathing can cause infants to not develop as they should since extra energy is being used for breathing instead of growing.[150] Nutritional issues are also associated with obstructive sleep apnea (described in further detail below, under Feeding).[128] Up to two out of three children with syndromic CS and multisuture CS have obstructive sleep apnea.[150]

- **Adenotonsillar hypertrophy:** This condition refers to having enlarged tonsils and adenoids, the structures toward the back of the throat that play a role in the body's immune response. Adenotonsillar hypertrophy is a key cause of obstructive sleep apnea. Removing both the tonsils and the adenoids can often resolve obstructive sleep apnea in typically developing children, but in those with CS, additional surgeries may be required.[150] Adenotonsillar hypertrophy occurs in 13 percent of children with any type of CS and is even more common in multisuture CS.[148]
- **Tracheal cartilaginous sleeve:** In this condition, the typical rings of cartilage that line the trachea (windpipe) are replaced with a sleeve of cartilage. This can cause the airway to be rigid and prevent adequate clearance of secretions. It has been found in up to 80 percent of children with syndromic CS, particularly those with Apert, Crouzon, and Pfeiffer syndromes.[103,151]
- **Chiari malformation:** This is a condition in which brain tissue extends into the spinal canal instead of staying within the skull. A Chiari malformation can impact the respiratory system since the brainstem contains the respiratory control center, which tells the lungs to breathe in and out.

Airway management at birth may include unique positioning of the infant to ensure the airway is open properly. Other management techniques may also include placing a nasopharyngeal airway device and the use of assisted ventilation.[152]

A nasopharyngeal airway device creates an open path for airflow when the airway space is constricted (see Figure 3.6.2). The device may be used temporarily after birth until surgical correction can be done.

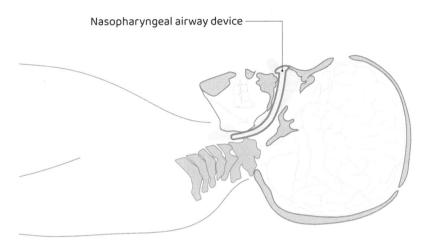

Nasopharyngeal airway device

Figure 3.6.2 View of nasopharyngeal airway device placement in an individual with Apert syndrome. Adapted with kind permission from John Persing, MD. Original image by Xioana Lu, MD.

Assisted ventilation is the use of an external device to help with natural breathing.[152] It can be noninvasive or invasive:

- **Noninvasive ventilation:** Examples include a continuous positive airway pressure (CPAP) machine or bilevel positive airway pressure (BiPAP) machine. A CPAP machine connects to a mask and provides continuous airway pressure to keep the airway open. CPAP is commonly used to treat obstructive sleep apnea. A BiPAP machine delivers high pressure and low pressure to mimic breathing in and out, which helps people who have challenges with effective breathing. Masks for CPAP and BiPAP machines may fit over the face, or for infants, just over the nose (referred to as nasal CPAP or BiPAP), as shown in Figure 3.6.3.

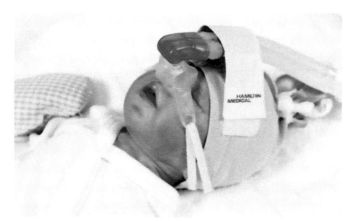

Figure 3.6.3 Infant with a nasal CPAP. Reproduced with kind permission from Hamilton Medical.

- **Invasive assisted ventilation:** This is done by placing a tracheostomy tube in the trachea (windpipe) through a small surgical opening. Figure 3.6.4 shows a child with a tracheostomy tube. The tube can bypass the area of restriction caused by midface hypoplasia or other structural abnormalities in individuals with syndromic CS. Ventilation devices can be connected to this tube to support breathing.

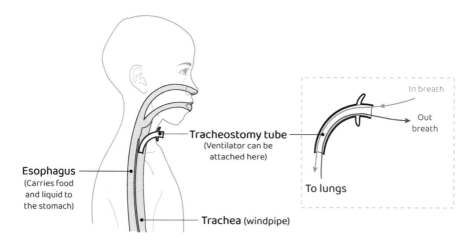

Figure 3.6.4. View of tracheostomy tube placement in a child. The tube can be connected to a ventilator to provide assisted ventilation.

Airway issues may resolve once structural conditions, such as mid-face hypoplasia, are corrected, or they may persist. If they do resolve, interventions such as tracheostomy tubes may no longer be needed and can be removed.

Feeding

Infants born with syndromic CS may have difficulty feeding because of the abnormal airway development and structure. Feeding and swallowing are often affected in those with Apert, Crouzon, or Pfeiffer syndrome.[153] This can result in malnutrition, as one study found in 44 percent of individuals with syndromic CS or multisuture CS.[150] Infants with syndromic CS are at a high risk of obstructive sleep apnea, which can increase their risk for malnutrition.[150] In addition, as the infant grows, the commonly observed atypical positioning of the jaw and teeth in syndromic CS may make chewing difficult.

Feeding may be managed with nutritional interventions, such as supplementing feeding with high-calorie shakes by mouth or liquid nutrition, either through the nose or through a surgical opening in the stomach.[154] There are three placement options for feeding tubes:

- **Nasogastric tube (NG tube):** inserted through the nose to carry nutrition to the stomach.
- **Gastrostomy tube (G-tube) (also called "PEG" or "percutaneous endoscopic gastronomy tube"):** surgically inserted into the stomach.
- **Jejunostomy tube (J-tube):** surgically inserted into a section of the small intestine (jejunum).

An NG tube is considered a short-term nutrition option. If nonoral feeding is expected to last longer than six weeks, a G-tube or J-tube is typically recommended. Of the three options, G-tubes are the most common and are typically preferred over J-tubes because they allow the food to enter the body at an earlier stage in digestion. G-tubes can also supply a large quantity of food at once, and more quickly, compared to the slow drip feeding used with a J-tube.

Some children with syndromic CS will need a feeding tube only for the short term until structural issues can be corrected. Others may need to rely on a tube for the long-term.

Eye closure

Eyelids serve as covers, keeping out debris from our eyes, preventing infection, and preventing damage from the sun or other harmful irritants. But the eyelids of infants with syndromic CS may not close completely, putting them at risk of damage to the cornea and vision impairment or loss[93,63]

The eyes of infants with syndromic CS are affected due to midface hypoplasia and the lack of forehead growth. Normally, a person's eyes sit within bony sockets (orbits) designed to keep them at a depth that allows the eyelids to close properly. When the socket shape or depth changes, the eyes may either sink back in or, more commonly, protrude or bulge out. This can make the eyelids ineffective at protection because they may not be able to cover the eyes.

When infants are born with severely bulging eyes and are not able to close them, a surgery called tarsorrhaphy may be needed. In this surgery, the eyelids are sewn partially together. This may be done temporarily until the infant is able to undergo CS surgery.[153] Other eye surgeries may also be needed shortly after birth to protect the eyes from permanent damage.[63,102]

Cognition, behavior, speech, and language

If you can't fly, then run. If you can't run, then walk.
If you can't walk, then crawl, but whatever you do,
you have to keep moving forward.
Martin Luther King Jr.

Cognition and behavior

Cognition and behavior issues vary in presentation and severity with syndromic CS. If present, they can affect a child's ability to actively participate in their medical care, recovery, therapy, and long-term outcomes.

Intellectual disability may be diagnosed in childhood or adolescence if it appears there are deficits in intellectual functioning measured by IQ;[*] adaptive skills such as communication, social skills, and independence; and school functioning.[83,155] The impact of syndromic CS on intelligence appears to be syndrome dependent:

---

[*] The broad average range of IQ scores in a typical population is 85 to 115. An IQ score of 70 or below indicates intellectual deficits.[82,83]

- There is a higher probability of being diagnosed with an intellectual disability with Apert and Muenke syndromes than with Crouzon or Saethre-Chotzen syndromes.[156]
- Those with Pfeiffer syndrome types 2 and 3 often have severe developmental delays and intellectual disabilities.[93]

Studies of behavior and related areas of functioning indicate that problems in these areas appear to be syndrome dependent:

- Apert, Muenke, and Crouzon syndromes are associated with higher rates of social and attention problems compared to the typical population.[156]
- Muenke syndrome is associated with an increased risk of behavioral and emotional issues compared to other types of syndromic CS.[109,156]

Knowing children with syndromic CS are at an increased risk of cognition, behavior, and related issues can help with monitoring and intervention, though signs of delay may not be apparent until a child starts school.[51] To help identify and better understand specific concerns, a referral for a neuropsychological evaluation can be helpful. Neuropsychology is a specialty that focuses on understanding brain functioning as it relates to cognition and behavior.[87] A neuropsychological evaluation provides an individualized assessment of the skills and abilities that are linked to coordinated brain functions such as memory, cognition, perception, problem-solving, and verbal abilities. Concerns related to these skills and abilities may indicate developmental delays. Neuropsychological testing can also be valuable in identifying individual strengths and needs, assisting with securing additional resources and interventions, and following progress over time or changes after interventions.

Speech and language development

Individuals with syndromic CS may have issues related to speech and language development due in part to hearing loss.[90,91,131] A contributing factor may be the presence of a submucous cleft palate (a specific type of cleft palate), which affects approximately three out of four individuals with syndromic CS.[148] Unlike a cleft palate, the roof of the mouth in an individual with submucous cleft palate appears intact but the muscles underneath are not formed properly. Submucous cleft palate may cause issues with speech and language development.

Speech and language development appears to be syndrome dependent. Children with Apert, Crouzon, and Pfeiffer syndromes often have anomalies that impact several areas of speech, including pronunciation of words and language development.[153] Referral to a speech and language pathologist (also termed "speech and language therapist") is recommended for individuals with syndromic CS.

Key points Chapter 3

- Syndromic CS usually has a genetic cause and is part of a syndrome (a syndrome is a group of characteristics that consistently occur together). Syndromic CS accounts for 15 percent of all CS cases.
- There are almost 200 syndromes associated with CS. Five of the most prevalent are Apert, Crouzon, Pfeiffer, Muenke, and Saethre-Chotzen.
- Syndromic CS often involves the premature fusion of multiple sutures.
- Increased intracranial pressure, hydrocephalus, and Chiari malformation occur in individuals with syndromic CS at higher rates than in those with nonsyndromic CS and may require treatment or additional surgeries, such as the placement of a shunt to treat hydrocephalus.
- Airway management, feeding, and eye closure are initial management concerns in individuals with syndromic CS and may need to be addressed prior to surgical repair of CS.
- Syndromic CS may be accompanied by concerns related to cognition, learning, and behavior. These may result in intellectual disabilities and developmental delays. These are generally more prevalent in children with syndromic CS compared to children with nonsyndromic CS.

Chapter 4

Surgical management and treatment of craniosynostosis in infancy

Introduction

And once the storm is over, you won't remember how you made it
through, how you managed to survive. You won't even be sure
whether the storm is really over. But one thing is certain. When you
come out of the storm, you won't be the same person who walked in.
That's what this storm's all about.

Haruki Murakami

The treatment for prematurely fused sutures in CS is surgical repair.
For *nonsyndromic* CS, typically a single surgery is all that is needed in
infancy (i.e., before one year of age). For *syndromic* CS, surgeries are
often required both in infancy and sometime later at different ages (see
Chapter 7).

This chapter describes common surgeries for correcting CS in infancy
and provides a general overview of what to expect. The timing and
technique of each surgery may vary among surgeons and hospitals.
The craniofacial team is the best resource for specific information
about surgery.

USEFUL WEB RESOURCES

Preparing for surgery

Before anything else, preparation is the key to success.
Alexander Graham Bell

The medical team

The preparation for surgery begins several weeks ahead of the surgery and involves the craniofacial surgeon, neurosurgeon, and other specialists on the team. They will evaluate the infant for any potential issues that may affect surgery.

A medical professional, typically a pediatrician, will do a physical exam and take a preoperative history. As well, as the child will be undergoing anesthesia, an anesthesiologist will do an evaluation that includes discussing family history of any issues with anesthesia, any bleeding disorders, and any cardiac or respiratory concerns.

An infant with CS may also be referred to an ophthalmologist prior to surgery to be examined for eye abnormalities.[54] They will look especially for papilledema, which is swelling around the optic nerve that may indicate increased intracranial pressure.

Other specialists may be needed before surgery for those with syndromic CS, such as otolaryngologists, who specialize in ears, nose, throat, and airway. Table 4.2.1 summarizes typical specialist visits that infants with CS may need prior to surgery.

Table 4.2.1 Specialist visits prior to surgery for infants with CS

SPECIALIST	AREA OF EXPERTISE	FOCUS FOR CS SURGERY
Pediatrician	General childhood growth and development	• Preoperative history • Physical exam
Anesthesiologist	Evaluation, monitoring, and care before, during, and after surgery while delivering anesthesia.[157]	• Family history of problems with anesthesia • Blood loss and need for blood transfusion • Pain control during and after surgery
Ophthalmologist	Eyes and vision	• Protection and correction of eye issues • Detection of papilledema
Otolaryngologist	Ears, nose, throat, airway	• Airway; need for tracheostomy, other airway interventions and management

Note: Surgery for individuals with *nonsyndromic* CS will likely involve only the first three specialists (pediatrician, anesthesiologist, ophthalmologist). Surgery for individuals with *syndromic* CS will likely need all the listed specialists.

The family

Each hospital has its own practice, and it's important for the family to ask any questions they have about the surgery planned for their child. Preparing for surgery can be overwhelming. These points may help:

- Many parents find it helpful to keep a notepad handy to write down questions that come up in the days before surgery, on the day of surgery, and during the hospital stay.
- Some hospitals, especially those who care for infants and children, will offer the opportunity to take a tour before surgery, which can

help lessen stress on the day of surgery. Parents can ask questions about the stay, such as who can visit and when, what comfort items to bring along (stuffed animals, special blankets, etc.), what food is available, and any other room-related questions. If an in-person tour is not an option, ask about a virtual or video tour, which many hospitals offer.

- Child life specialists are frequently available in children's hospitals and can work with children in age-appropriate ways to prepare them for surgery. Child life specialists can also provide siblings strategies that may be useful to prepare them for what their brother or sister will look like after surgery, particularly if siblings will be visiting in the hospital.

- The child may need to be bathed and have their hair washed with special soap the day before or the day of surgery, following specific instructions from the hospital. This is done to help prevent infection.

- Specific instructions on when the child needs to stop eating and drinking will be provided. It is important that these be followed exactly. To ensure the child does not have access to any food or drink after that time, it's recommended that parents check the car seat and back seat area of their vehicle for stray food or bottles before leaving for the hospital, especially if the child is old enough to grab items and put them in their mouth independently.

Surgical repair

You never know how strong you are,
until being strong is the only choice you have
Bob Marley

The history of CS surgery goes back to the first known corrective procedure in 1890 done by French surgeon Odilon Lannelongue.[158] Early surgeries involved releasing or removing the affected suture through an open incision. However, outcomes were poor and the procedure was discontinued. It wasn't until the 1920s, with advances in surgical technique and medicine, including blood transfusions, that a successful surgery to remove the affected suture was performed.[158,159]

CS surgery is an area of continual development. Currently, it is done by one of two methods, both described in detail in this section:

• **Endoscopic surgical repair:** Skull bones around the fused suture are cut and the suture is removed through small incisions in the skull, but no extensive skull bone remodeling is done.
• **Open surgical repair:** Skull bones, including the suture, are cut and/ or removed and remodeled.

These methods may be used for both syndromic and nonsyndromic CS. If there is a particular concern about increased intracranial pressure being present at birth, such as may occur in syndromic CS, an initial surgery may be done to relieve and prevent the immediate pressure.[61] Syndromic CS may also require additional CS surgical repair after infancy if the sutures progressively fuse or re-fuse.

Timing of surgical repair

When the craniofacial surgeon is planning CS surgical repair, there are two main factors they consider: the timing (the age of the child when the surgery will be performed) and the type (which sutures are affected), and one depends on the other. Some types of CS may be corrected earlier, while others are better corrected later.

The craniofacial surgeon, in consultation with the multidisciplinary team, will ultimately determine the timing and type of the surgical repair to achieve the best outcomes, both immediate and long-term. In making that decision, they will consider the infant's age and size (history of prematurity, developmental concerns), type of CS and sutures involved, family history of bleeding or clotting disorders or anesthesia complications, presence of increased intracranial pressure or a Chiari malformation, and other factors.

There is no consensus on the optimum age for surgical correction, but most craniofacial surgeons agree it should be done before the child's first birthday, as surgical repair done after the age of 12 months has been associated with higher surgical complications.[160] In general, the younger the infant, the greater the potential for natural brain growth to help reshape the skull and for the bony gaps from surgery to heal.[161] In addition, the bones of the skull begin to ossify (harden) and become less moldable as the infant grows. This is why older infants will require the open method of surgical repair.

Endoscopic surgical repair is usually performed between two and four months of age.[3,27,62] This type of surgical repair was first used for sagittal CS repair and is a widely accepted treatment for this type of CS. Emerging data suggests that endoscopic surgical repair of metopic, coronal, and lambdoid sutures is also successful in infants two to three months of age. Continued evaluation of long-term outcomes is needed.[162,163] Endoscopic surgical repair is always accompanied with helmet therapy afterwards.

Open surgical repair is usually performed later than endoscopic surgical repair and can be done at different ages. In one recent large-scale review of research, open surgical repair was reported as a safe option in young infants, including those younger than six months of age.[164]

Table 4.3.1 provides a summary of the timing for both surgeries. **Note:** Not all possible options are included, and practice is continually evolving. Parents should discuss any questions and concerns related to specific surgical techniques with the craniofacial surgeon.

Table 4.3.1 Timing of surgical repairs

SURGICAL REPAIR	TYPE OF CS	TYPICAL AGE OF INITIAL SURGICAL REPAIR
Endoscopic	Nonsyndromic Syndromic (as an initial repair)	• 2 to 4 months[3,27,62]
Open	Nonsyndromic Syndromic	• 4 to 12 months[128,164] • Initial surgical repair may be earlier or later in syndromic CS • In childhood and beyond, if needed

Endoscopic surgical repair

An endoscopic surgical repair is less invasive compared to open surgical repair. It is associated with less time in the operating room, shorter hospital stays, less blood loss, and lower overall medical costs.[165,166,167] However, the family and child must adhere to prescribed helmet therapy consistently after surgery. The percentage of infants having endoscopic surgical repair for any type of CS increased from 4 percent in 2014 to over 13 percent in 2019 in the US.[167] Not all centers offer endoscopic surgery.

In this repair, the surgeon uses a camera to visualize and work through one or two small incisions. Specialized tools are used to release and cut the bone and remove the affected suture. Additional cuts may be made, but no extensive remodeling is done.

Simply removing the suture does not correct the shape of the skull, however. Correcting the atypical head shape will depend on helmet therapy after the surgery.

Figure 4.3.1 illustrates the sequence in endoscopic surgical repair when used to correct sagittal CS. The early timing of this surgery—often between 6 and 12 weeks of age, but no later than 4 months[3,7,27,62]—allows for the natural growth of the brain to help reshape the skull with helmet therapy.[161]

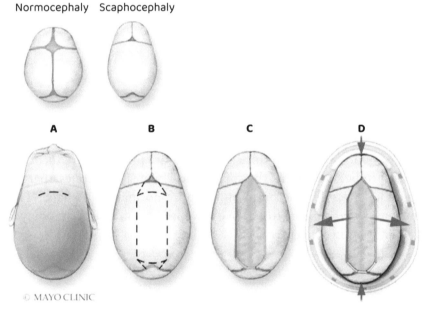

Figure 4.3.1 Infant skull without CS (normocephaly; top left) and one with sagittal CS (scaphocephaly; top right). Steps in endoscopic surgical repair with helmet therapy for sagittal CS repair (bottom). **A:** Small cuts are made in the scalp (dashed lines). **B:** Skull bones around the closed suture are cut. **C:** Skull bone and fused suture are removed. **D:** Helmet is worn after surgery for skull reshaping. The arrows indicate the direction of skull growth after surgery. Used with permission of the Mayo Foundation for Medical Education and Research, all rights reserved.

Helmet therapy after endoscopic surgical repair helps correct the shape of the skull. The helmet, or helmet orthosis, is custom-made so the protruding part of the head is confined while open areas are left to allow for growth that will produce a symmetrical head shape. Helmet orthoses are usually made of lightweight, plastic or carbon fiber (see Figure 4.3.2). The helmet is worn 23 hours a day for several months until the desired skull shape is achieved, typically until the child is at least 12 months. Because the brain and skull grow rapidly in this period, the helmet will need to be adjusted frequently.

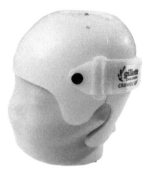

Figure 4.3.2 Helmet orthosis.

Another technology that can be paired with the endoscopic approach is the use of surgical springs to shape the head instead of a helmet. After the abnormal bone is removed, springs are placed where the fused bone used to be. Over time, the springs slowly push the bones apart to create more space for the brain and a more normal head shape. This requires a second surgery to remove the springs, and the technology is not available at every center.

Open surgical repair

Open surgical repair is done through a larger incision compared to an endoscopic surgical repair. It involves remodeling of the bones, not just removing the affected suture.

The goal of open surgical repair is to increase the cranial vault volume and make more space to accommodate the growing brain. The cranial vault is the space that encases and protects the brain. This repair for CS is generally referred to as cranial vault remodeling (CVR). Several techniques may be used, depending on which sutures are involved. The basic principle of each repair is the same; the cranial bones are cut and/or removed, reshaped, and often secured with resorbable plates and screws. (Resorbable plates and screws are composed of materials that break down and are absorbed into the body, so they don't have to be removed.)

Open surgical repair produces more immediate results compared to endoscopic surgical repair and does not require helmet therapy afterwards.[7] However, it is a longer surgery, requires a longer hospital stay, more frequently requires blood transfusions, and costs more.[165,166,167]

Different open cranial vault remodeling surgical repair techniques are described.

a) Posterior cranial vault remodeling

Posterior cranial vault remodeling addresses areas at the back of the head and is typically used to correct lambdoid CS (see Figure 4.3.3). The occipital bone of the skull is removed, reshaped, and put back in place with resorbable plates and screws. This surgical repair is typically done at four to six months of age.[5]

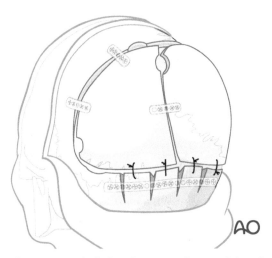

Figure 4.3.3 Skull showing posterior cranial vault remodeling for lambdoid CS. AO Surgery Reference, www.aosurgery.org. Reproduced with kind permission. Copyright by AO Foundation, Switzerland.

b) Anterior cranial vault remodeling with fronto-orbital advancement

Anterior cranial vault remodeling addresses areas in the front of the head. This is typically performed with the fronto-orbital advancement surgical repair, which corrects the supraorbital rim and upper eye socket area by moving the forehead forward.

Figure 4.3.4 shows a skull view following fronto-orbital advancement in a child with metopic CS. The remodeled forehead improves eye protection and reshapes the eye sockets. Typically, this is used to correct metopic CS, unicoronal CS, and bicoronal CS, and is usually done after six months of age.

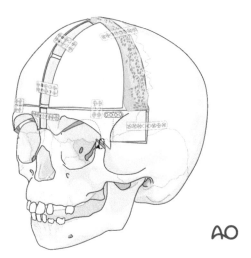

AO

Figure 4.3.4 Skull showing fronto-orbital advancement. AO Surgery Reference, www.aosurgery.org. Reproduced with kind permission. Copyright by AO Foundation, Switzerland.

c) Near-total cranial vault remodeling

Near-total cranial vault remodeling, also known as a midvault remodel, addresses both the front and back areas of the head. It may be used to correct sagittal CS, and it is typically done between four and eight months of age. Figure 4.3.5 shows a near-total cranial vault remodeling in a child with sagittal CS.

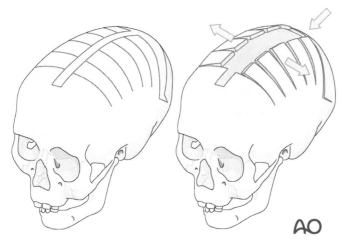

Figure 4.3.5 Skulls showing near-total cranial vault remodeling. AO Surgery Reference, www.aosurgery.org. Reproduced with kind permission. Copyright by AO Foundation, Switzerland.

d) Total cranial vault remodeling

A total cranial vault remodeling also addresses both the front and back areas of the head. This is commonly used to correct multisuture CS, for reoperations, or for repair in older children. It is typically done after six months of age. See Figure 4.3.6.

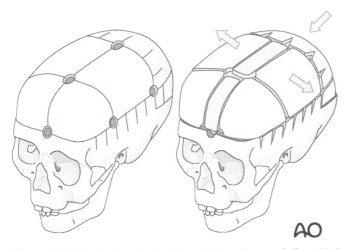

Figure 4.3.6 Skulls showing total cranial vault remodeling. AO Surgery Reference, www.aosurgery.org. Reproduced with kind permission. Copyright by AO Foundation, Switzerland.

e) Cranial vault distraction osteogenesis

Another open surgical repair is distraction osteogenesis ("osteogenesis" means "formation of new bone").[168] This technique is used for multisuture syndromic CS and has historically been done in infancy. It involves creating cuts in the skull bones and inserting a device that slowly pushes the bones apart each day while the body creates and lays down new bone in the open space. After the surgery and hospital discharge, the parents manually turn the inserted device at regular intervals, typically twice per day, with a small tool. Each turn pushes the bones apart at a fixed rate.

Figure 4.3.7 shows a posterior cranial vault expansion using this technique, showing the tool inserted between the bones that have been separated. This technique may be used in other parts of the skull and face, including for an anterior cranial vault expansion, which pushes out the front of the skull. Timing of this surgery varies and depends on the surgical goals.

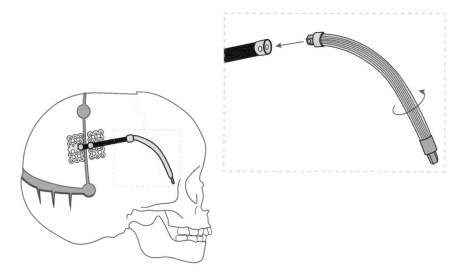

Figure 4.3.7 Lateral view of skull showing posterior cranial vault expansion by distraction osteogenesis. The tool disconnects from the device when not in use. Pink lines show where the bones have been separated. Adapted with kind permission from AO Foundation, Switzerland.

Keegan had a total cranial vault remodeling done for sagittal and partial lambdoid craniosynostosis when he was just past 16 weeks of age. Even though technically he had more than one suture fused, his craniosynostosis was considered nonsyndromic.

You might think because I work in the medical field I would do a vast amount of research on what surgery entails, but I took the opposite approach; I didn't want to know specific details about the actual surgery until it was done. My husband felt similarly, knowing that handing Keegan over to skilled craniofacial surgeons was for the best. If this is how you are feeling, just know you are not alone. It is okay to not want a lot of details and to just focus on the outcome. After the surgery was over, we were ready to hear about the exact details of the surgery and were amazed with every step. If you do want more details about the surgery, make sure you ask your craniofacial surgeon to explain their approach to you, as simply or as complicated as you would like.

Risks

Risks associated with CS surgery have decreased significantly over the last several decades. Major complications are rare: the rate of morbidity (temporary or permanent disability) is 5.0 percent and the rate of mortality (the number of deaths that occur due to a specific illness or condition) is 0.1 percent for most high-volume craniofacial centers.[62]

Two of the most common risks include:

- **Blood loss and blood transfusion:** Blood loss is common in CS surgery, and frequently infants require a blood transfusion, although recent advances have decreased this need.[169] Smaller infants will have less blood volume, so losing blood can be more concerning for them than larger infants.[170] Blood transfusions are needed in 19 percent of endoscopic surgical repairs and 62 percent of open surgical repairs.[167]
- **Anesthesia:** Anesthesia can present risks to infants and small children due to their smaller airways, less developed organ systems, and increased challenges with maintaining body temperature.[171,172]

Additionally, rare but serious complications may occur, which may result in brain damage.[51,173]

- **Cerebrospinal fluid leak:** A leak of fluid that surrounds the brain and spinal canal.
- **Stroke:** A condition when a blood vessel in the brain is either blocked or ruptured.
- **Air embolus:** One or more bubbles of air become trapped in blood vessels.
- **Infection:** An infection occurs at the surgical site or in brain tissue.

Later complications after surgery include nonideal wound healing and irregularities in the skull shape. It is estimated that persistent bony defects after open remodeling occur in 5 to 20 percent of cases, necessitating an additional surgery.[62] Correction of these is described in Chapters 6 and 7.

Parents should discuss specific questions and concerns about the risks of surgery with the craniofacial team.

> Keegan needed a blood transfusion during and just after surgery, as well as three days after surgery.

Reducing surgical risks

Practices to reduce CS surgical risks[*] include:

- Reduce the need for blood transfusions.
  - Medication (epoetin alfa) and supplements (iron) may be given for three weeks prior to surgery to increase the infant's circulating red blood cells. This has been shown to decrease the need for blood transfusions during and after surgery.[174,175]
  - A medication (tranexamic acid) may be administered during surgery to improve the blood clotting mechanism. This has been

---

[*] The practices listed are those in place at Gillette Children's at the time of the writing. Each medical center will have its own practices.

shown to decrease the volume of transfused blood that is needed and decrease the need for blood transfusions.[128,171,175]

- o A craniofacial surgeon and a neurosurgeon may perform CS repair together, in a dual surgeon approach. This allows for a shorter operative time and less time under anesthesia. Longer operative times are associated with greater blood loss.[175]
- Prevent infections
  - o Warming measures may be implemented approximately 30 to 60 minutes before surgery and continued throughout surgery to keep the infant's temperature within the normal range and prevent hypothermia. This has been shown to prevent surgical site infections as well as minimize blood loss.[171,172,176]
  - o Administration of antibiotics* has been shown to decrease surgical site infection rates.[177]
- Minimize postoperative scar appearance and prevent hair loss
  - o Meticulous and immediate hemostasis (stopping the bleeding) may be done as the incision is made rather than using surgical clips on the scalp to stop the bleeding. Surgical clips may cause damage to the hair follicles, increasing the occurrence of hair loss (alopecia).[178]

Keegan looked so tiny in his crib in the recovery room. He had a white dressing wrapped around his head with a small drain tube coming out behind his left ear, as well as multiple wires and IVs (intravenous lines). We were transferred to the pediatric intensive care unit later that day, and by evening, I was able to hold him, which was the best feeling in the world! He would cry whenever he was moved, but this improved over just a couple of days. He definitely slept best when I held him.

When he was awake, he was enamored with the oxygen saturation monitor that was attached to his toe, as it had a red light on it, and he would follow it with his eyes whenever he moved his foot. We were prepared that his eyes might swell shut over the first few days, but he had minimal swelling, and his eyes were open the whole time. We had brought a photo with us of what he looked like before surgery and

---

* A specific antibiotic protocol is followed as recommended by the Children's Hospitals' Solutions for Patient Safety, which is a collaboration of pediatric hospitals in the US and Canada. This protocol specifies which antibiotics should be given and when.

hung it on the wall, so everyone could see what he looked like without swelling. Everyone loved Keegan's big smile in the photo.

There were many visits from the medical team making sure Keegan was comfortable and progressing well after his surgery. Child life specialists met with us and brought different items for us to use during our stay, including a mobile with fish that moved across the screen that Keegan found entertaining. The nurses went above and beyond to make sure Keegan stayed comfortable during his recovery as well. They stayed on top of his pain medication the first few days, and each one was very helpful and answered the many questions we had about the safest way to hold him, feed him, and how to care for his incision.

During his stay, three professional athletes came to visit children in the hospital and hand out autographed photos and memorabilia. Keegan looked like he was going to cry when they were in our room, so I said it was because he was probably getting hungry. The biggest and tallest of the athletes quipped, "I can relate to that!"

Keegan smiled for the first time two days after surgery when the surgeon removed the dressing. That's when I knew Keegan was still the same bright and happy baby he had always been, but now he had a beautifully shaped head to match.

When Keegan was sleeping or my husband was holding him during our hospital stay, I worked on making ribbons for prayer chains to send to the Cranio Care Bears organization, who would then send them in care packages for other kids with craniosynostosis before their surgeries. I made ones that said, "For when I am weak, then I am strong," a Bible verse from 2 Corinthians 12:10, which has helped us through this craniosynostosis journey. My other quote was from Bob Marley, "You never know how strong you are, until being strong is the only choice you have."

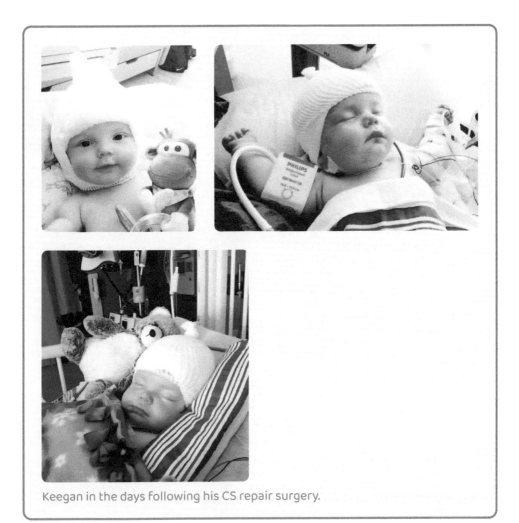

Keegan in the days following his CS repair surgery.

Recovering from surgery

Scars show us where we have been.
They don't have to dictate where we are going.
David Rossi

Recovery will depend on the type of surgery done, as well as on the individual child and the hospital. Hospital stays often disrupt sleep and feeding routines, and it may take a couple of weeks to get back on schedule. It's helpful to anticipate the recovery period after surgery, including caring for the child and what family support is in place for parents and other family members. Typical recovery expectations are outlined below.

Endoscopic surgical repair

Endoscopic surgical repair generally requires less time under anesthesia and has a shorter recovery period compared to open surgical repair, with a hospital stay of just two to three days. Keeping the surgical area clean and protected from injury is important. Helmet therapy is generally started one to two weeks after surgery and continues until the child is at least 12 months of age.

Contour irregularities (bony irregularities) that feel like small bumps and lumps on the skull may occur, although these are less likely compared to open surgical repairs.

Postoperative follow-up visits with the craniofacial surgeon will be needed.

Open surgical repair

Open surgical repair is more extensive than endoscopic surgical repair and generally requires a longer recovery period. Due to the larger incision and longer time in the operating room, swelling in the face and head is typical. It is common for the eyes to swell shut a day or two after surgery, but this will gradually improve.

Keeping the surgical area clean and protected from injury is important. To avoid sun damage and improve the long-term appearance of scars, the child should always wear a hat when in the sun. Helmet therapy is not required.

Contour irregularities (bony irregularities) are expected. These may feel like small bumps and lumps on the skull and may occur anywhere on the skull (not just near the incision). They may occur with endoscopic surgical repair as well, but not as commonly. They should resolve on their own within a year or two as the body makes new bone to fill in the irregular areas and heal. If they persist, a smaller surgical repair, a cranioplasty, may be done to smooth them out (see Chapters 6 and 7 for further details).

Post-operative follow-up visits with the craniofacial surgeon will be needed.

Pain management

It is normal to be concerned about pain after surgery. Since most CS surgeries occur during infancy, the child may not be able to verbalize when they are experiencing pain. It may be difficult to determine whether they are crying due to pain, hunger, nausea, or other reasons. Often, pain assessment in infants and young children is done by watching for certain behaviors. Common indicators of pain in infants and children include:[179,180,181]

- Crying, screaming and/or moaning
- Complaining of pain
- Being irritable, whiny, crabby, or showing negative behavior
- Being inconsolable (cannot be calmed)
- Not being comforted by distractions
- Inability to sleep or very restless, fitful sleep
- Having a change in muscle tone, usually with increase in muscle tightness or spasms
- Not being able to find a comfortable position
- Holding very still, seeming to guard against touching or moving areas of the body that had surgery
- Being unwilling to play or take part in routine or favorite activities
- Showing a change in usual behavior (e.g., an active child being quiet or withdrawn)
- Showing a change in appetite; poor intake of food or liquids

Each craniofacial team will have specific pain management practices. The goals of pain management are to minimize pain and help the child rest so they can heal and return to normal activities. Medication and nonmedication therapies may be used.

Medications including opioids and non-opioids may be used.[182] Opioids can be obtained only with a prescription and are typically given for a short duration after surgery, usually 24 to 48 hours. Examples are morphine (given only in the hospital) or oxycodone (may be given at home). Usually, they are not needed once the child goes home, though each child will be different.

Non-opioids are medications that can be purchased over the counter and do not require a prescription. These may be taken for a longer period after surgery. Examples are acetaminophen and ibuprofen.

Nonmedication therapies may include activities such as resting and keeping the head elevated during sleep. Distracting the child with a book, music, or other activity may also help.

After we returned home from the hospital, we were ready to stay on top of pain medication but were amazed at how quickly he recovered. He had opioid pain medication only one day at home, then he did well with over-the-counter pain medicine. He was happy anytime he was upright, such as being held or in an infant seat, but when we tried to lay him flat in his crib he would cry. It was probably about two weeks before we were able to have him lie flat without him fussing. His temperament was unchanged after surgery. He was an overall happy baby who loved to babble on and on for hours and still does to this day—anyone who knows him will attest to that!

Having Keegan go through surgery shortly after I returned to work added a bit more to the stress level. I had taken a 12-week maternity leave, the maximum amount I was able to take, and Keegan had his surgery when he was four months old. I requested a week off from work to help care for Keegan after his surgery because I wanted to have more time with him, and I didn't have any more vacation time available.

My parents played a huge role in supporting us by watching our older son during the many doctor appointments, surgery, and hospital stay. They were our go-to people if we needed any help once we returned home from the hospital as well. When we did return home, our house was clean and snacks and meals were prepared for us—such servant hearts they have! My sisters were also on the top of our list if we needed extra hands.

My husband and I had talked to our daycare provider about Keegan's surgery. We shared what we felt would be expected during recovery, primarily keeping him away from other children to protect his head, as well as possible pain medication needs. Our daycare provider owned an in-home daycare and was so supportive and reassuring to us. Keegan was able to return to daycare without any issues. And after a few weeks, our neighbor's daughter who had babysat the kids in the past began to watch him for us again without any difficulties.

Keegan's incision went over the top of his head from ear to ear. We joked that his head looked like a baseball with the stitches. It was amazing how quickly the incision healed. As he became more mobile and learned to crawl and walk, anytime he bumped his head we would be so worried, but he would be completely unfazed and would continue his merry way. For example, he would stand up while under a table and whack his head, and we'd run over to him expecting him to be crying in pain, but he'd just get up and walk away like nothing ever happened. I've always said his head is stronger than all of ours!

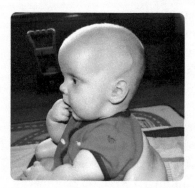

Side view of Keegan and his surgical scar.

Key points Chapter 4

- The treatment for CS is surgical repair.
- Most children with nonsyndromic CS will need a single operation sometime before their first birthday.
- Children with syndromic CS will often require more than one surgery.
- Collaboration with other specialties is needed as well, especially for syndromic CS, and the child may see several team members.
- Surgical repair of CS may be either endoscopic (a less invasive surgery done through small incisions with specialized tools) or open (removal and remodeling of the skull bones through a larger incision).
- The type of surgical repair selected is based on the age of the child at diagnosis as well as the type of CS.
- Risks of surgery include the need for blood transfusion, risks associated with anesthesia, and other more serious risks such as cerebrospinal fluid leak, brain damage, stroke, air embolus, infection, or very rarely, death.

Chapter 5

Deformational plagiocephaly

Introduction

Pick your baby up.
Pick your baby up.
Pick your baby up.
Martin Lacey

Deformational plagiocephaly (DP), also referred to as positional plagiocephaly or occipital plagiocephaly, is the change in shape and flattening of an area on the head that occurs due to *external* forces. The head shape that results may look like CS, as described in section 2.5, but it is *not* CS.

DP is different from CS in several respects:[183]

- DP is a change in head shape from forces occurring *outside* the skull: CS is a change in head shape from a force occurring *inside* the skull.
- DP is *not* caused by premature fusion of the cranial sutures; CS *is* caused by the premature fusion of the sutures.

- DP is most often treated by physical therapy, positioning, and helmet therapy; CS is treated surgically; it cannot be treated by helmet therapy alone.

DP is the most common cause of an atypical head shape in infants, with the prevalence estimated to be as high as 20 to 50 percent in six-month-old infants.[7] Most often, it occurs on the back of the head from the infant frequently lying on their back. It can also affect the side of the head if the infant prefers to look toward one side more than the other for prolonged periods. When DP predominantly affects the side instead of the back of the head, it is often described as right-sided or left-sided DP, and the ear on the side of the flattened area shifts forward along with the base of the skull.[184] DP is treatable with conservative treatments and does not require surgery. After treatment, a typical life can be expected.

Note that an infant can have DP *together* with CS. Treatment of DP and CS at the same time can present challenges and requires a craniofacial surgeon experienced in both conditions.

Figure 5.1.1 shows the skulls of three infants: one typical, one with DP affecting the back of the head, and one with DP affecting the right side of the head. Note how the right ear and forehead shift forward in the infant with right-sided DP. Note also that, in contrast to CS, the sutures in infants with DP remain open. The altered head shape is unrelated to the sutures.

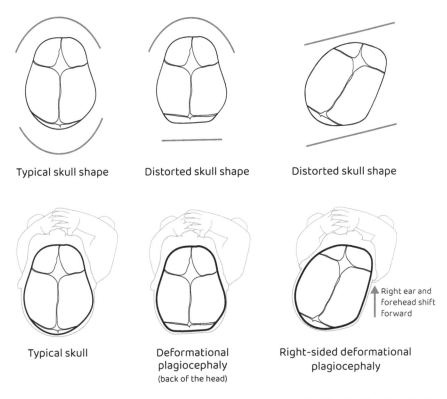

Typical skull shape   Distorted skull shape   Distorted skull shape

Typical skull   Deformational   Right-sided deformational
                     plagiocephaly   plagiocephaly
                    (back of the head)

Right ear and
forehead shift
forward

Figure 5.1.1 Superior views of infant skull: typical shape (left); DP affecting the back of the head (middle); right-sided DP (right).

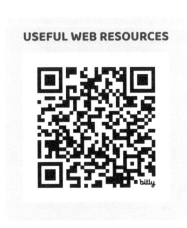

USEFUL WEB RESOURCES

Causes and risk factors

I alone cannot change the world, but I can cast a
stone across the water to create many ripples.

Mother Teresa

Both causes of and risks for DP are different than CS, and therefore
treatment is different.

Causes

DP is caused by external forces that change the shape of the skull. The
force causing the condition can happen before or during the birth (20
percent of cases) or after the birth (80 percent of cases).[7]

After birth, this external pressure is the result of how the infant is positioned. That is, if an infant is consistently placed in a specific position,
the area experiencing the highest pressure may become flattened over
time.[185] For instance, using car seats, bouncy seats (bouncers), and
strollers (push chairs) results in infants lying or reclining on their backs

with their heads in constant contact with the surface behind them. Extended periods of time in these devices can lead to DP.[186]

Despite this concern for DP, which may in part be due to infants sleeping on their backs, experts strongly recommend always placing infants on their backs for sleeping. This advice originated from the Back to Sleep campaign,[*] introduced in 1992 in the US to address the rise in cases of SIDS (sudden infant death syndrome).[†] The main premise of this campaign is that "back is best," and that infants should be put to sleep only on their back, on a firm surface with no soft objects or loose bedding. The campaign was successful in decreasing the prevalence of SIDS in the US by more than 40 percent.[188,189] However, the increase in positioning infants on their backs also led to a significant increase in DP[185,190,191,192]—from approximately 5 percent in the early 1990s[192] to 20 to 50 percent in the 2000s.[193]

Risk factors

Risk factors for an infant developing DP include:

- **Male sex:** It is estimated that males are up to three times more likely than females to be diagnosed with DP.[2]
- **A multiple pregnancy:** Having twins or triplets (or more).[185]
- **Being firstborn:** A study of infants with DP found 61 percent were firstborn.[191]
- **Breech position:** The baby lying bottom or feet down in the uterus.[191,194]
- **Prolonged labor with assisted delivery:** This includes the use of forceps and vacuum-assisted delivery.[185,192,191]
- **Prematurity:** Infants born prematurely are at higher risk of having external forces push on and shape their head while the bones are still hardening.[195] Premature infants are more likely to need to spend time in the NICU (neonatal intensive care unit) to receive specialized care immediately after birth and less time being held.[196] This will increase the time the infant's head is in a fixed position.[2,197]

---

* The Back to Sleep campaign (later expanded to Safe to Sleep) is endorsed by the US National Institute of Child Health and Human Development, American Academy of Pediatrics, World Health Organization, and Centers for Disease Control and Prevention.

† SIDS is "the sudden death of an infant under one year of age that remains unexplained after a thorough case investigation."[187]

Premature infants also often prefer to lie with their head turned to one side consistently.[198]

- **Congenital muscular torticollis:** This condition describes the persistent shortening of one of the sternocleidomastoid (SCM) muscles.[199] The term "congenital" means this condition is present from birth. In infants with DP, 15 to 20 percent have neck muscle imbalance, or torticollis, though it may be underreported and underdiagnosed.[7,200] The big SCM muscles are on each side of the neck. They provide head tilt and rotation and help with pointing the chin downward. When the SCM on one side is atypically tight, the infant will prefer to turn their head in one direction over the other, often resulting in DP. Figure 5.2.1 shows an infant with a left-sided contracted (shortened) SCM resulting in left sided torticollis. This infant shows a preference to turning their head to the right, which as can be seen in the posterior view, results in right-sided DP (the flat area on the back of the head is on the right side).

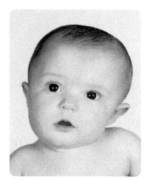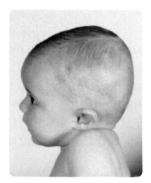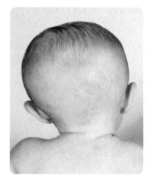

Figure 5.2.1 Infant with left-sided torticollis and right-sided DP: anterior (left), lateral (middle), posterior (left). Images provided courtesy of Cranial Technologies, Inc.; © Cranial Technologies, 2024.

Treatment

Life is from the inside out.
When you shift on the inside,
life shifts on the outside.
Kamal Ravikant

Treatment for DP aims to address the forces that caused the altered head shape in the first place and to implement measures to help mold the head back to a more symmetrical appearance. When parents are provided education and strategies right after birth, DP can often be prevented, or its severity lessened.[201] Early detection and intervention have been shown to have the most positive impact on correcting DP, likely because the skull is most moldable during periods of rapid growth, which is highest in the first year of life.[186,202]

In some children, DP may resolve on its own as they grow or be less noticeable as hair growth begins.[203] The rate at which DP resolves on its own is not known, and there is no good predictive model to determine which children will have an atypical head shape without treatment. If DP is left untreated or incompletely treated, especially when it is severe, it may result in atypical skull shape and facial asymmetry, affecting the child's appearance.[203] It may also be difficult to find head gear and helmets that fit well (such as cycling helmets or those required for sports).

There are three treatments typically used for DP: repositioning, physical therapy, and helmet therapy. The goal of each is to improve head shape. Which treatment is best is challenging to report because there is no standard classification system to measure improvement. The outcome often depends on the severity of the DP—mild, moderate, or severe. This is a subjective rating system determined by clinical examination and based on visual inspection.[203] Some objective measures do exist, using measurements of the infant's head taken directly or from images or models.

Often, parental satisfaction with head shape is used as an outcome measure. Where possible, we have included outcome data for each of the three treatment types.

Repositioning

Repositioning (sometimes referred to as counterpositioning) is the easiest and most recommended first step to correct DP. It is particularly useful if DP is noticed in the first few months of life, before helmet therapy is appropriate. Repositioning is more effective in resolving DP in infants younger than four months of age,[202] and it is done at home by the parents, often under the guidance of a physical therapist.

The most common area where DP occurs is at the back of the head; therefore, increasing the time infants spend lying on their stomachs (tummy time) or sides, while supervised, can be an effective treatment.[183] Daily repositioning and planned tummy time should be encouraged for at least 30 minutes spread over 24 hours.[204,205] In addition, holding the infant and using approved carriers rather than always placing them in strollers or infant seats can be effective.

If an infant strongly prefers to look to one side, there are simple techniques that parents can use to help encourage them to move their head to the other side. Placing objects for the infant to look at on the other side, holding or feeding the infant so the other side is facing outward, and moving the crib or changing the environment to encourage the infant to turn their head can be helpful.[186,192,206,207]

Repositioning is often effective until the infant can hold their head up independently, turn side to side on their own, and sit unsupported. These skills are generally mastered between four to seven months of age; after that, repositioning is generally not effective.[185,208]

Physical therapy

Physical therapy may be recommended to learn some of the repositioning techniques and teach muscle-strengthening exercises. Physical therapy leads to better head shape results compared to repositioning education alone, plus outcomes can be achieved in a shorter period, especially for severe DP.[209]

Using physical therapy as a treatment for DP that is not accompanied by torticollis involves education and repositioning techniques. The frequency of appointments may vary, but the repositioning techniques should be used throughout the day by the parent at home.

Physical therapy is particularly important when DP is accompanied by torticollis. When it begins early, it can be effective.[210] The exercises need to be repeated several times every day at home by the parent and continued until the torticollis is resolved. A typical recommendation is to do the exercises with each diaper change. Generally, the younger the infant starts physical therapy, the shorter the time is needed to resolve the torticollis.[186]

Helmet therapy

Helmet therapy for DP was first introduced in 1979.[211] It is widely used in many countries to treat moderate to severe DP, or when repositioning and physical therapy have failed to show improvement.[186,209]

Modern technology and new materials have improved the fitting and wearing of helmets.[210,212] Today, helmets can be created using a 3D digital model of the child's head, which allows for a custom fit. The helmet is constructed to allow for growth that will produce a symmetrical head shape.[210] Figure 5.3.1 shows an infant during the 3D scanning process to fit a helmet.

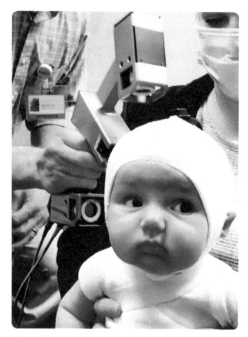

Figure 5.3.1 Infant being scanned for helmet fitting using 3D process.

Figure 5.3.2 shows the outline of a head inside a helmet, showing where growth is expected and where the helmet will restrict growth.

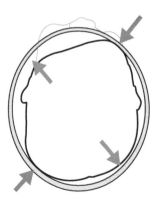

Figure 5.3.2 Image of head inside helmet used for treatment in DP (yellow outline). Teal arrows show expected growth; orange arrows show where the helmet will restrict growth.

Once the child starts helmet therapy, it is important they follow the schedule for wearing it. For best results, this typically means wearing it almost full time, usually 23 hours a day. The helmet will need to be adjusted as the child's head grows. This is typically accomplished by space from the inside of the helmet being carved out as the head grows, often allowing the same helmet to be used the entire time.

Helmet therapy for DP is not painful; minor skin irritation is the most common concern. Other complications may include temporary hair loss or incomplete (or inadequate) correction. Close monitoring for skin issues and ensuring the helmet is evaluated and adjusted as prescribed helps.[210]

The ideal age for helmet therapy is between four to eight months of age. The child will typically need to wear the helmet for 3 to 6 months, generally stopping therapy after 12 months of age when the skull growth slows.[192] Figure 5.3.3 shows an infant undergoing helmet therapy.

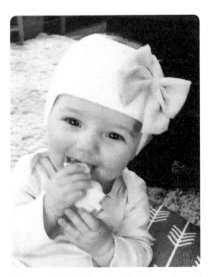

Figure 5.3.3 Infant with DP undergoing helmet therapy.

When the helmet is worn consistently, complete correction of DP is achieved in 94 to 96 percent of infants.[213] In addition, improved facial symmetry and aesthetics are achieved with helmet therapy.[214,215,216]

Figure 5.3.4 shows an infant's head with right-sided DP before and after helmet therapy.

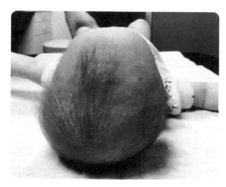 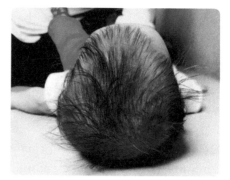

Figure 5.3.4 Superior views of a child with right-sided DP before (left) and after (right) helmet therapy.

Disparities in access to care exist in the treatment of DP. Helmet therapy is expensive and the resources to create the helmets are not available everywhere. Children from lower-income backgrounds are more likely to present for treatment later and not receive helmet therapy.[217] In addition, some parents may choose not to pursue helmet therapy due to the commitment to the intense wearing schedule.

Families should discuss helmet therapy with the craniofacial team.

Key points Chapter 5

- Deformational plagiocephaly (DP) is the change in shape and flattening of the head that occurs due to external forces exerted on an area of the head for a prolonged time. It is not CS though may be confused with CS, and may even occur *with* CS.
- Positioning the infant in a consistent position (typically on their back) is a common cause of DP.
- Prevalence of DP has increased since 1992 in the US due to the Back to Sleep campaign.
- Treatment for DP includes repositioning, physical therapy, and helmet therapy. Unlike treatment for CS, treatment for DP is *not* surgical.

Chapter 6

Growing up with nonsyndromic craniosynostosis

Introduction

A butterfly does not return to a caterpillar after it is mature.
We must learn to grow and evolve into a stronger, wiser,
and better version of ourselves. Life occurs in stages and
taking a step at a time is key to learning and growing.
Kemi Sogunle

Most often, children with nonsyndromic CS require a single surgery, prior to their first birthday, to resolve CS. The growth and development of the child's skull and face need to be monitored by the craniofacial surgeon for several years after surgery, typically until about five to seven years of age. As well, some children may need annual eye exams to continue to monitor for signs of increased intracranial pressure.[20] Follow-up visits with the craniofacial surgeon will include evaluating for any symptoms that may indicate that the sutures have re-fused. Such symptoms include headaches, nausea, unusual sleep patterns, or abnormal development. Among children who have had CS repair (both nonsyndromic and syndromic), 33 percent may experience headaches.[218] Any issues with cognition, behavior, and speech and language should also be discussed during follow-up appointments. See section 2.6.

If parents have concerns about their child as they grow or worry that a symptom may be related to the CS, it is appropriate to reach out to the craniofacial surgeon to discuss. It's common for parents to be concerned about their child playing sports or participating in other activities. That concern and anxiety can increase depending on the intensity and amount of contact involved in the sport.[219] However, once fully healed from surgery, most children with nonsyndromic CS can participate fully in sports and activities without restrictions. The risk of a sport-related traumatic brain injury in a child with repaired nonsyndromic CS appears to be the same as in the typical population.[220]

"Health-related quality of life" (HRQOL) refers to the way in which a condition affects a person's well-being.[221] Children with nonsyndromic CS (surgically repaired) age 7 to 16 years have a similar HRQOL compared to typical children. Further, neither their CS type nor surgical method influenced HRQOL.[221]

USEFUL WEB RESOURCES

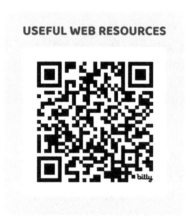

Additional surgery

Scars are tattoos with better stories.
Susan Stoker

Once surgically repaired, over 90 percent of children with nonsyndromic CS will not require any additional surgeries.[218,222,223] Most often, the initial surgical correction improves the shape of the skull and corrects facial asymmetries to a satisfactory level, and any remaining asymmetries are often not noticeable. A review of a number of studies shows general satisfaction with appearance following single suture repair surgery.[224]

Surgical correction aims to correct asymmetry as much as possible; however, it is important to note that the human face is not fully symmetrical even in the absence of CS. Small differences are not easily noticed and, in fact, perfectly symmetrical faces are not as visually pleasing as mildly asymmetrical ones.[225]

While children with nonsyndromic CS rarely require additional surgeries to correct asymmetry, bony irregularities may exist, and a surgery known as cranioplasty may be performed. This surgery is typically much less invasive than the original surgery, as the goal is to smooth irregularities as opposed to completely remodeling the bones. Irregularities can be smoothed using a bone substitute material. If larger corrections are needed, prosthetic implants can be used.[62] Cranioplasty to correct irregularities in the skull shape is typically done later in childhood, generally after age six.[3]

Keegan had routine checkups in the years after his surgery, and the surgeon confirmed it would be okay for him to participate in sports as he became older. The craniofacial team cleared him for any sport he was interested in and said craniosynostosis would not hold him back from doing what he wants to do. Keegan has tried a variety of sports and activities, including baseball, basketball, flag and tackle football, swimming, hiking, biking, sledding, ice skating, four-wheeling, and more—pretty much everything a young boy enjoys doing!

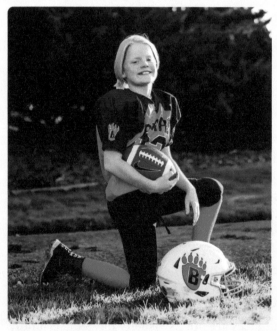

Keegan enjoys playing football, among other sports

Keegan is now a thriving 11-year-old. If you were not already aware of his journey, you would not guess that he is different from any other 11-year-old. Throughout childhood, he met all the developmental milestones without difficulties, likely from trying to keep up with his older brother. He has done well in school. His head shape receded a bit since surgery, but not to the level of needing another surgery. He graduated from clinical follow-up visits at seven years of age and has had no long-term effects.

We have talked about his surgery openly with him since he has been old enough to understand, and he will proudly tell anyone who asks about his scar all the details, to the best of his knowledge.

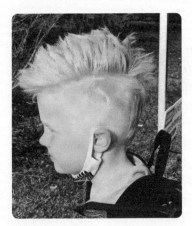 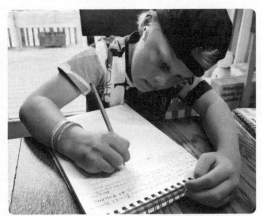

Keegan, age nine (left) and working on his story for this book (right).

Hi my name is Keegan Comstock I am 11 years old. And I was born with craniosynostosis. at 4 months old. But I don't remember surgery But I remember the checkups. The doctors were very nice and caring and I got to cross the skyway and look through the binoculars. And I remember the last appointment like yesterday and I was sitting waiting for the doctor to come in the room I then I figured out it was our last checkup and I was seven. I was sad and happy that i was sad coage I couldn't have time like that with my mom but im not sad anymore because i can have more. What I was is to tell peope that are about to have the surgery but not be embarressed with your scar.

Keegan's story in his own words.

> Hi my name is Keegan Comstock. I am 11 years old. And I was
> born with craniosynostosis. At 4 months old [I had surgery] but
> I don't remember the surgery. But I remember the checkups. The
> doctors were very nice and caring and I got to cross the skyway and
> look through the binoculars. And I remember the last appointment
> like yesterday and I was sitting waiting for the doctor to come in
> the room and then I figured out it was our last checkup and I was
> seven. I was sad and happy that I was sad because I couldn't have
> time like that with my mom, but I'm not sad anymore because
> I can have more time with my friends and family. What I want
> is to tell people that are about to have the surgery is to not be
> embarrassed with your scar.

Though Keegan's surgery and recovery went without a hitch, there have
been many times when craniosynostosis-related symptoms have crossed
my mind. He has had more headaches* in his adolescence than my first
child did, and I would wonder if it was craniosynostosis related or just
coincidence. The headaches became frequent enough that it prompted
us to make an appointment with the craniofacial team to discuss. They
asked us to continue to monitor the headaches as it did not seem to be

---

* Headaches may be a sign of increased intracranial pressure and should be reported to the craniofacial surgeon for evaluation. Follow-up appointments will likely include questions about the
occurrence and frequency of headaches.

craniosynostosis related at that time. The headaches began to lessen to the point where he rarely has headaches anymore.

Going through a journey like this definitely leaves an impact, and I do not feel it is uncommon for craniosynostosis families to question if certain things are related to craniosynostosis or not. If in doubt, always contact your craniofacial team to find answers. They will determine if further workup is needed or, at minimum, will put your mind at ease reassuring you that your concern is unrelated.

This was the hardest thing my husband and I had ever faced. Finding support along the way was the biggest factor that got us through it. We would not have been able to handle it if we didn't have such an amazing craniofacial team who gave us the time we needed and answered the many questions we had.

I do not recommend relying solely on your own Google research or social media groups for advice, because everyone's situation is different, and nothing compares to the many hours and years of dedicated teachings the craniofacial teams must go through. Their recommendations and expertise are priceless.

I believe going through hard journeys in life builds character and strength, whether by chance or by choice. Craniosynostosis became a passion my husband and I chose to embrace, and as a way of giving back to the amazing craniosynostosis community who helped us through our journey, we wanted to support others stepping into their journey. We started our own 5K walk/run, aiming to spread awareness to other craniosynostosis families and the community as a whole. We decided to hold the race the last weekend of June each year, as Keegan's surgery was at the end of June. We started it in 2013 with five "Cranio Warriors" attending with their families. The race is held in White Bear Lake, a suburb outside of Saint Paul, Minnesota (Keegan's 5K for Craniosynostosis Awareness (google.com)). In more recent years, we have had over 25 Cranio Warriors attend (some from out of state) and over 175 participants (family, friends, local community members). This race has provided more than just a fun morning of events; it has become a support system for all the craniosynostosis families who have helped each other through the years and who continue to welcome new families and help them along their journeys.

As Keegan and the other kids around his age are becoming older, the race is helping build confidence about having the scars on their heads. Instead of fearing what others may think, they embrace their scars as reminders of how strong they have been and how strong they continue to be.

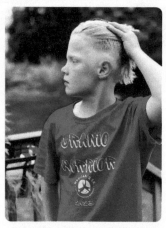

Keegan at the 2023 Keegan's 5K for Craniosynostosis Awareness.

On the ribbons we make for care packages, I now write, "Scars are tattoos with better stories." I still have the small bottle of body wash the clinicians asked us to use on Keegan's head after we were discharged from the hospital, and smelling it brings back a flood of memories and tears. The memories also flood back each year at race time as we put up signs for each of the Cranio Warriors along the running route. Seeing their hospital photos and current photos brings such joy to our hearts. We are so grateful for the craniofacial team who led the way in this journey. Now when we look back at the photo of Keegan's head when he was first born and see the heart shape, we understand how much really came from that heart.

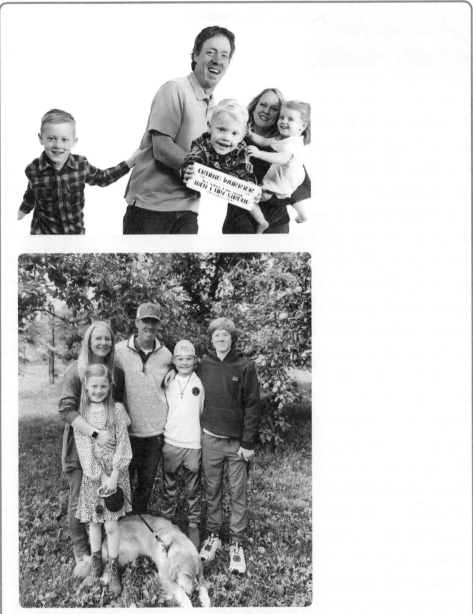

Keegan and his family. Back row, left to right: Mom (Heather), Dad (Jason), Keegan, Brayden. Front row, left to right, Eliza, Cooper.

Key points Chapter 6

- Ongoing follow-up of the child's condition continues until they reach about five to seven years of age, or beyond, if needed.
- Small differences in facial asymmetry may persist and should be discussed with the craniofacial surgeon if there are concerns.
- When needed, a surgery known as a cranioplasty may be done to address bony irregularities.
- Children with nonsyndromic CS have a typical health-related quality of life, and no major differences have been noted compared to children without CS.

Chapter 7

Growing up with syndromic craniosynostosis

Introduction

We are very much at the mercy of circumstance,
but it is how you choose to respond to
circumstance that determines the quality of your life.
Chris Matakas

The overall management of syndromic CS is complex and lifelong. This book focuses on the CS aspects of these syndromes; addressing other aspects is beyond the scope of this book. Further information on syndromic CS is included in **Useful web resources**.

- After surgery, the craniofacial surgeon will monitor the growth and development of the skull and face. Follow-up visits with the surgeon will include evaluating for any symptoms that may indicate that the sutures have re-fused, such as headaches, nausea, unusual sleep patterns, or atypical development. Among children who have had CS repair (both nonsyndromic and syndromic), 33 percent may experience headaches.[218] If parents are concerned about their child as they grow that a symptom may be related to their CS, they should contact the craniofacial surgeon.

- Any issues with cognition, behavior, speech, and language should be discussed at follow-up appointments. (See section 3.7.) In the US, accommodations may be made, such as an individualized education program. Frequent surgeries and recovery from those surgeries may affect school attendance. Parents are encouraged to keep in close communication with the school on the specific needs of each child.
- Annual eye exams with dilation are recommended to monitor for increased intracranial pressure.[20]
- Those with syndromic CS may be limited in what sports and other physical activities they are able to participate in.[215] This will vary greatly from one child to another and may change over time. The recovery time required for the multiple surgeries required may also interfere with participation in competitive sports. Children with syndromic CS should be encouraged and supported to participate in any sports and activities they are interested in and able to take on. Some modifications and specialized plans may be needed for sports and school participation.

USEFUL WEB RESOURCES

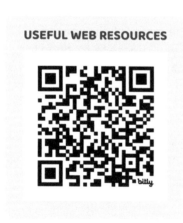

Additional surgery

Yesterday is gone. Tomorrow has not yet come.
We have only today. Let us begin.

Mother Teresa

Children with syndromic CS are more likely to need additional CS surgeries throughout their life. These may include repeat surgeries, staged surgeries, and surgery to correct irregularities in the skull.

Repeat surgeries are required if sutures re-fuse or progressively fuse as the child grows. One study reported that 31 percent required repeat surgery.[222]

Surgeries to address other aspects of CS may be planned for later in a staged fashion. Midface hypoplasia is typically first addressed between 7 to 12 years of age once the midface growth is nearly complete.[226] This may be done using the distraction osteogenesis technique (see Chapter 4) to improve the position of the cheek bones, bones of the midface, and sometimes the airway. A second surgery is frequently needed in the teen years.[61] A final surgery to correct dental issues and improve facial symmetry of the upper and lower jaw is completed after skeletal maturity, typically between 17 to 21 years of age.

A cranioplasty to smooth skull irregularities using a bone substitute material may also be needed. If larger corrections are needed, prosthetic implants can be used.[62] Cranioplasty to correct irregularities in the skull shape is typically done later in childhood, generally after age six.[3]

Because of the complex nature and involvement of many areas of the body of children with syndromic CS, other surgeries are also often needed, besides those for their skull or face. These may include:

- Eye surgery
- Syndactyly repair
- Cleft palate repair
- Dental and orthodontic surgery

Ideally, some surgeries will be performed together to decrease the number of times a child needs to be under anesthesia. A specialty craniofacial center that can coordinate the various aspects of care needed for children with syndromic CS is recommended. Further discussion of these surgeries is beyond the scope of this book. Additional information is included in **Useful web resources**.

Key points Chapter 7

- Ongoing follow-up for individuals with syndromic CS will likely continue throughout childhood and into adulthood.
- Individuals with syndromic CS may need additional surgeries throughout their lifetime. These may include surgeries to address CS as well as for other areas of their body.
- Individuals with syndromic CS may have difficulties in some sports and activities due to physical limitations or from the amount of time spent recovering from surgeries. Participation in activities should be encouraged and supported as much as possible. Some modifications and specialized plans may be needed for sports and school participation.

Chapter 8

Living with craniosynostosis

> Nobody gets to live life backward.
> Look ahead—that's where your future lies.
>
> **Ann Landers**

In this chapter, people share stories of living with CS, both nonsyndromic and syndromic CS, and one is from a family whose child had deformational plagiocephaly. The stories come from families who are early in their journey as well as those whose children had surgery many years ago. They are the voice of the parents and of an adult living with CS.

Raising a child with a condition such as CS is a journey, and each individual and family will have different needs. Understanding the journeys of others, as described in these stories, may be helpful, but don't judge your own journey against others.

Sheila, mother of four-year-old Evelyn, from Minnesota, US

Evelyn was born with unicoronal craniosynostosis. We noticed right away she had one eye that looked more open than the other. My husband, Brian, thought something was wrong. I just thought because she was breech she was a bit squished inside for so long that it would take a little while to straighten out. The nurses seemed to agree that it would get better in the days after her birth, but we didn't see much change.

At her five-week well-child check, the pediatrician felt a ridge on her skull above her left eye that ran down toward her ear. She had also developed a flat spot on one side of the back of her head. After discussing this with the pediatrician, we decided to take Evelyn to see a craniofacial surgeon to make sure everything was okay. On the way to that appointment, we thought in the worst-case scenario she would need a helmet. We had no idea what we were in for!

Evelyn had a CT scan that showed her sutures were fused, causing one of her eye orbits to be misshapen and her skull to be held back. This news was so scary and devastating. I felt a lot of guilt about things I had done during my pregnancy: Did I have too many chocolate shakes while pregnant? Did this happen because I opted to stay on my antianxiety medication? I also blamed myself for *not* doing some things. The baby had been breech, and I should have been more active. I thought maybe because she was stuck, her head grew wrong! I should have tried to get her to turn more. No matter what anyone said, I really felt deep down that I caused the problem.

I tried to take Evelyn to a new-baby class, but the questions from other moms about diapers and burping just felt so small compared to what I was dealing with. I didn't want anyone to know she had an issue. We didn't even share the diagnosis with extended family right away, as we didn't want people to pity our beautiful new daughter. I wanted to protect her from that.

We had to wait until she was six months old for surgery. The anxiety of waiting during this time was really difficult. I just wanted the surgery over so her poor little brain wouldn't be squished in her skull. I also kept staring at her perfectly beautiful head. It was hard to believe there was a problem underneath the beautiful skin. I didn't want to believe that my husband and I created something that was flawed. I didn't want anything to change for her. She was beautiful the way she was to me.

Between the time of Evelyn's diagnosis and shortly after her surgery, I found it helpful to write about our journey to share with select family and friends through an online blog. We were also able to get connected with other parents who had been through this journey before, and they were so helpful in answering my questions.

Some excerpts of my blog posts help to convey my stress and feelings of anxiety as we neared the surgery day.

> Surgery is only 12 days away. We got some information about the surgery from a nurse yesterday…preparations, what to bring, what to expect. The call lasted a good 30 minutes and was very overwhelming. This mama is feeling anxious. Mainly I don't want her to get sick before surgery so we don't have to postpone. The

waiting has been hard. Luckily, I have a rock-solid hubby and a sweet little two-year-old to hug me all day long. The dog lies by us for protection and support, too.

———

Surgery is six days away. I'm very worried about Evelyn getting sick and having to postpone. I have decided to quarantine us for the remainder of the week to minimize exposure. It would really stink to have to wait another few weeks after waiting five months for this surgery. This mama's heart could not handle it. I keep thinking of the surgeon's words telling me that she will look different and will have lumps and bumps for the next year or so. It will take a little while to get used to. I am in a bit of mourning over her beautiful head which right now is smooth, perfect, and scarless.

———

Tomorrow is the day. We have to be at the hospital early in the morning. Her surgery will last three to four hours and after that she will spend the night in the pediatric intensive care unit (PICU). Send up some prayers for us in the morning. I took a picture of her beautiful head of hair. I'm hoping it will grow back fast. I'm trying not to think about tomorrow, but it's all I've been thinking about for a long time. Other moms I have talked to who have gone through this have mentioned the feeling of relief once the surgery is over. I cannot wait for that feeling and to be on the other side of this.

Day of surgery

She is out. I'm holding her as she sleeps, hoses and all. She looks pale and her voice is hoarse. But she is ok.

The surgery Evelyn had was a cranial vault remodeling with a fronto-orbital advancement. It went well, and she had her first haircut by the surgeon! I was so relieved when I was able to hold her afterwards, even though she had so many lines coming out of her tiny body.

The day after surgery

Today she is a little swollen. They say she will look swollen for the next three weeks. She can still open her eyes, so that's good. She will need a blood transfusion today. There were a lot of alarms going off overnight, mostly with her moving around and kicking. The best thing that happened overnight was the 4 a.m. party. Evelyn threw it for herself... babbling and kicking and playing with toys. It seemed like the old Evelyn was back. This morning she has been enjoying snuggles and sleeping on mom and dad. She is so sweet. I'm hoping she will want to drink milk again soon. She did eat oatmeal for me. These things take time, they say.

Two days after surgery

No more drains!* Yay! Evelyn is detached from everything and only has one IV needle taped to her right hand. She started to nurse again. Woohoo! She is doing well with her pain and swelling. She has been sleeping great, although staying in the hospital can mix everybody's nights and days up. I'm so grateful and proud today. Evelyn has handled this whole thing with such grace. We have a lot to be thankful for.

Three days after surgery

Home! Evelyn did so well that we got to take her home this morning. Her stitches are dissolvable so that is good. We have a follow-up in three weeks and then again in about six months. We are so happy that things will return to normal. We have to keep her big brother careful and gentle around her, but overall we're back to normal. Amazing.

---

* Surgical drains may be used following surgery. They are small plastic tubes/devices to collect fluid from around the incision area (draining it instead into the tube). Most are removed two to three days after surgery.

Two weeks after surgery

We have been home for a while now and Evelyn is healing nicely. She does have some lumps and bumps, but she is overall cheerful and off all pain medicine. She is back to eating solid foods, but her sleep is back to newborn status; awake every two to three hours. Evelyn does not want to sleep without being held right now, understandably. It makes for a tired mama.

Evelyn's recovery continued without any issues. At around age two, we had to bring her back to see the craniofacial surgeon because her head didn't seem to be growing much and she was having some problems sleeping. However, everything checked out okay and she has not had any other issues since.

Today, Evelyn is a happy, healthy four-year-old. She loves reading, dancing, princesses, music, art, and rainbows. She is highly coordinated and can already pedal a bike with no training wheels. She has done many things at an earlier age than her older brother did. She will need one last surgery to correct a couple of small areas on either side of her forehead. Small amounts of filler will be put in to even out the appearance of her skull. Luckily, this is a short, one-night stay and we will get this done before she starts kindergarten. She is amazingly optimistic and the toughest person we know.

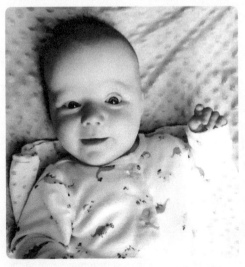

Evelyn, six months old, the morning of her surgery.

Éamon, father of 10-year-old Éanna, from Limerick, Ireland

We call Éanna our little miracle man.

We had been trying to have children for over eight years when Éanna was born. At that time, I was nearly 50 years old and Rosemarie was in her mid-40s. We had gone through the plethora of fertility treatments—IVF,* donor egg, etc.—to no avail and had all but given up hope of being parents. But then one day, a month or so before my birthday, Rosemarie walked into the house and announced she was pregnant. We were over the moon and bursting with excitement and anticipation.

The pregnancy was by and large a good one with regular scans showing no issues or concerns until week 18 when bleeding near the placenta was noticed and again at week 30. Our consultant physician informed us that the rate of growth had slowed and was not following the normal trajectory. She recommended a series of tests, including an amniocentesis (a test that collects a sample of the amniotic fluid that surrounds the baby during pregnancy), which caused some worry for us as it was used to screen for various syndromes.

Going through this was difficult for both of us. For me, the week of waiting for the results was the longest and most agonizing of my life, with little or no sleep and fearing the worst. Thankfully, these tests didn't identify any specific syndromes but still didn't explain the slowdown in growth. So, while there was a certain relief with the results, we were still beset with constant worry.

What followed next was weekly scans with close monitoring and eventually Rosemarie being admitted to the maternity hospital at 36 weeks pregnant. Éanna was born at 38 weeks gestation by cesarean section, weighing just 5 lb, 9 oz (2,534 grams). Seconds after he was born, I was allowed into the operating room where the cesarean section was performed and was relieved to hear the wailing of a newborn baby, one with a beautiful and angelic face. However, immediately we could see

---

* IVF, or in vitro fertilization, is a type of fertility treatment that is done by manually combining egg and sperm in a laboratory dish to create an embryo. The embryo is then transferred to the uterus.[227]

that Éanna's head was relatively small and odd shaped, having a long head, chin to top, as if he had a chef's hat on. Within hours of his birth, he needed to be transferred to the children's hospital where he spent the next 10 days undergoing all sorts of tests. His poor little foot was like a pincushion with all the blood samples he had to provide. However, through it all, when I looked at his little face, I sensed a resilience and a business-like attitude as we went from appointment to appointment. He was alert, engaging with his surroundings, and he bonded with me immediately (Rosemarie had to stay in the maternity hospital for medical reasons, and the separation was naturally very distressing). I instinctively sensed there and then that everything was going to be okay.

The tests revealed that Éanna had craniosynostosis. In Éanna's case, his type of craniosynostosis involved multiple sutures, namely the metopic, coronal, and sagittal sutures. The resulting skull shape was trigono-turry-brachycephaly. We learned that Éanna's craniosynostosis was most likely due to a gene mutation.

The doctors explained to us that craniosynostosis can affect a child's brain and development. If left untreated, it can lead to increased pressure in the skull and serious developmental problems, such as not being able to read and requiring intensive special education. (In that respect we have been very lucky as Éanna's remaining issues are primarily cosmetic.)

When Éanna was a few months old, Rosemarie enrolled him in an early-intervention program near our home where he continued for several years. This program helped with his gross and fine motor skills, speech, and general development. Éanna progressed so much that they recommended discharging him when he was seven years old. In fact, Éanna himself by then was questioning why he had to attend the sessions.

Éanna attends mainstream school and is just above the middle of the pack academically, which is exactly where we would like him to be, craniosynostosis or no craniosynostosis. In other aspects he has outperformed his peers, being able to both swim and ride a two-wheeled bike at just three and a half years old.

He has had three surgeries on his head: the first two were to create room for his brain to grow and the third was mainly cosmetic. It is only now that I can bring myself to read the detail of those operations. I deliberately chose not to know what was involved in the surgeries at the time. After each, his head was bandaged, his eyes were swollen, and his surgical wounds needed monitoring and cleaning.

Fortunately, the first two surgeries were completely successful. The third one achieved its objective in terms of reshaping his head, but it stretched his scalp too much and killed some hair follicles, resulting in a bald patch at the back of his head. A final operation, called "tissue expansion," is scheduled in summer 2024 to address this. If successful, we hope Éanna will be like any other young boy going into secondary school, both in appearance and intellect.

Éanna continues with regular monitoring for any impact on his eyes, ears, nose, and hormone levels. These regular follow-up appointments will continue until he is in his late teens.

Éanna is now 10 years old. Throughout the surgeries, follow-ups, and various other appointments, he has shown resilience and determination way beyond his years. He attends a great school with brilliant and caring teachers. One of our fears was that he would be bullied or teased because of his appearance, in particular the bald patch at the back of his head, but to this point that has not been an issue. He is very popular and has very good friends who know him as the soccer-mad little man with the hat! The odd time when he is outside his immediate familiar environment, some people have passed a remark, but his attitude has always been "It doesn't bother me. If they have a problem, it is their problem, not mine."

We are so, so proud of him, love him dearly, and are so thankful to have him in our lives.

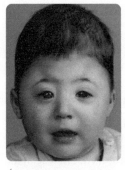 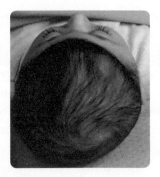 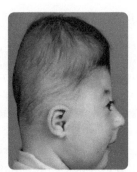

Éanna at six months of age.

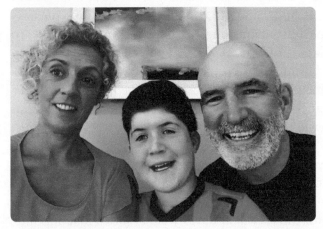

Éanna at 10 years of age with his parents, Rosemarie and Éamon.

Dulce, mother of 11-year-old Dulce Guadalupe, from Texas, US

Dulce Guadalupe, or DG, as we call her, was born with metopic cranio-synostosis. My pregnancy with her was uneventful; neither of her two older brothers had craniosynostosis. I knew immediately at birth that her head shape didn't seem right. It looked like an egg to me. I even asked the pediatrician, right after she was born, who reassured me it would go back to normal. Other things were troubling as well: she was a fussy baby, always crying, she barely napped, and she would wake up screaming as if she was in pain and nothing would calm her down. At her two-week well-child appointment, I brought up my concerns about her head shape but was again reassured it would go back to normal. Two weeks later, at her cardiology appointment (she was born with a benign heart murmur), the cardiologist could feel a ridge on her forehead and recommended I take her to another pediatrician to have it evaluated. At that appointment, it was decided she needed to have an MRI done. I felt relieved to be finally getting some answers.

DG was able to have her MRI done without any sedation; she just slept right through it after I nursed her. The results were sent over to a craniofacial surgeon who called me three days later to schedule an appointment for her for the very next day. I went alone to that appointment, as my husband had to work. When the craniofacial surgeon came into the room and told me that DG had metopic craniosynostosis and would need surgery, I felt tremendous sadness and started crying. I was so scared for my baby.

The hardest part was telling her big brothers about the surgery she would need. They were 5 and 11 at the time, so they were able to understand some of what was happening, but my husband and I didn't want them to feel as worried as we did. They were both heartbroken.

After we received DG's diagnosis, everything seemed to move quickly. She was six months old when she had her cranial vault remodeling surgery. The worst part was waiting the seven hours of surgery to hear that everything was okay. When we saw her after surgery for the first time, it was like seeing a different baby—her facial features had changed so much. It might sound weird, but I missed her "before-surgery face" so much.

She spent four days in the hospital before we were able to bring her home. For the first week or two, she didn't want to sleep without being held. Thankfully, after that she started sleeping through the night, and her crying fits were much less.

She recovered well from her surgery, but she started showing some issues with meeting her milestones. At nine months of age, she started receiving occupational, physical, and speech therapy to help with this.

When she was two and a half years old, she needed to have a surgery to reconstruct her eye muscles. This surgery went extremely well, without any issues. She's a rock star!

DG was eventually diagnosed with intellectual disability and speech impairment. Through genetic testing, we found out that she had a chromosome duplication that was responsible for her developmental delays and other problems. Every time I read anything about kids with metopic craniosynostosis thriving in all aspects of their childhood, I feel heartbroken for my sweet girl and all the struggles she is going through. We know her challenges will likely be lifelong, and it scares me to think about how she will manage as an adult.

When she was five years old, she needed to have a second cranial vault remodeling. Since she was older and able to understand more, we could prepare her ahead of time, and this surgery went very well. Around the age of eight, she had to have another eye muscle reconstruction surgery, which she also handled tremendously well. She is really the bravest person I know!

Today, DG is 11 years old and in the sixth grade. She receives special services at school to help her, and little by little she is reaching her milestones. She is a hardworking girl, and we are so proud of her. She has been one of the biggest blessings in our lives. We adore her kind, sweet, compassionate nature.

Her brothers were—and continue to be—amazing through all of this. They treat her with so much care and love. They also treat her no differently than if she did not have a disability. They have learned to see beyond that and see her beautiful soul, heart, and the amazing girl she is.

My advice to new parents starting this journey is to listen to your gut. If you feel something is wrong, do not stop until you get an answer to your concerns. We are the voice of our children and their biggest advocates.

DG has come a long way, and despite all the struggles she's had since she was a baby, she is happy, kind, and compassionate. I'm so happy she is ours and that God gave her to us.

Elaine, mother of four-year-old Senan, from Sligo, Ireland

In 2019, at just a few weeks old, our second son, Senan, was diagnosed with sagittal craniosynostosis. His head was unusually narrow from birth, and when I asked about this, various doctors and nurses reassured me that it was the result of "molding" in utero before birth. He had trouble with breastfeeding, and in an attempt to figure out what the issue was, I hired both a breastfeeding consultant and an osteopath.[*]

The breastfeeding consultant noted Senan's tense, tight jaw and again felt that the issue was the result of molding, which would resolve itself. The osteopath told me to check with the general practitioner, and I distinctly remember him saying that it was "not normal" but offered no other insights.

We had an appointment with a consultant pediatrician when Senan was four weeks old for an unrelated matter, and again they reassured us that the head shape was unlikely to be problematic, with a "99 percent sure" comment, which was reassuring at the time. Nevertheless, Senan was scheduled for an X-ray in subsequent months. There was no apparent sense of urgency at that point.

At the six-week check with our family general practitioner, things changed. While he had no prior experience with this type of case or concern, he urged me to follow up immediately with the hospital. The

---

[*] An osteopath is a doctor of osteopathic medicine, someone who follows a whole-person approach to health and wellness.

look in his eyes made me a little afraid. For the next few days, I rang the hospital insistently and was informed that there was some confusion about the type of scan required and that they would get back to me soon.

A few days later, Senan collapsed unexpectedly in my arms after a feed in what turned out to be what medics refer to as "an unexplained, resolved, medical event" rather than anything related to the early fusing of his skull bones. We rushed him to emergency, and after triage, various examinations, and lengthy discussions with the physician on call, he was admitted, which gave quicker access to an X-ray.

Over the next few days, Senan had more than one X-ray, along with an EEG and an MRI. One of the consultants explained to me that there was a possibility that his skull bones had fused early, and they would need to refer us to a children's hospital in Dublin.

A few days later, we made the trip to Dublin where a CT scan confirmed a diagnosis of sagittal craniosynostosis, a term we were not familiar with. We were presented with options for surgery, and despite the risks involved, we consented in order to give our boy the best possible chance in life. We were referred to the craniofacial team at the children's hospital and put on a list for surgery to take place when Senan would be approaching six months of age. The most valuable advice I received at this time was from a public health nurse who encouraged me to take care of myself both physically and mentally, and to do what was needed to get through.

In the days, weeks, and months before the surgery, I often felt highly anxious. As the surgery date neared, I isolated myself from the outside world. However, the moment I handed my baby over to the nurse to carry him to the operating room at the hospital, I felt an odd sense of relief. Things were now officially out of my hands—I would have to place my full trust in the medical team. Happily, the surgery was a success, and after six weeks of recovery, our little baby boy began to thrive and develop.

As a parent, I was hungry for facts and evidence throughout this journey. I asked many questions of the medical team and read a great deal in relevant medical journals. I learned how to pronounce the terminology and about the different surgery options available to us. I knew the statistics for mortality risk, brain injury, and other complications that might result from the surgery. I joined social media support groups and got to know other parents of children with similar diagnoses. They provided both practical support—what personal items we may want to take to the hospital, what to wear, and so forth—as well as emotional support and reassurance.

Planning the logistics of the trip to hospital and surgery was important for me: booking accommodation, packing our hospital bags, organizing Grandma to come and stay in our home with our elder son (then six years old). It was impossible to shelter our elder son completely, and he did show some changes in his behavior. We offered him certainty where we could, telling him, for example, "Mummy and Daddy will leave on Tuesday morning. Grandma will pick you up from school on that day." Being a psychologist, I encouraged him to talk about or draw how he was feeling, putting a color on the feeling if possible (red for anger, yellow for worry, blue for sad, and green for calm/happy). My husband and I answered questions as simply and honestly as we could, without going into detail about things he didn't need to know. We did not make promises we could not keep. Now he only vaguely remembers those experiences.

There were a lot of emotions for us to process in the months after Senan's surgery, and seeking opportunities to write or talk helped us to make sense of them. I am extremely grateful to the incredible cranio-facial team in Dublin and all our family and friends who supported us through a very challenging period.

Senan will have follow-up appointments until he turns 15 years old for routine reviews and to assess the potential for more surgery. However, we focus our attention on day-to-day family living and feel blessed to have two healthy, resilient sons who continue to bring fun and adventure to our lives.

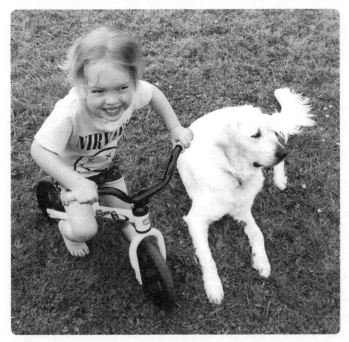

Senan, age three, and his dog Sailor.

Leah, mother of eight-year-old William, from Minnesota, US

I didn't know anything about craniosynostosis when I was pregnant with my first child, William. During my pregnancy, I developed pre-eclampsia, a pregnancy condition that is accompanied by high blood pressure and excess proteins in the urine. Once this was diagnosed, I needed ultrasounds every other week to check on William. Despite the frequent ultrasounds, the craniosynostosis was not discovered prenatally and everything appeared normal during my pregnancy.

Around 34 weeks, I developed HELLP syndrome, a life-threatening condition that is often a progression of preeclampsia. Many times, delivery is needed. Since the hospital I was scheduled to deliver at did not have a neonatal intensive care unit (NICU), and it was looking like William would be born prematurely, I was sent by ambulance to a specialty hospital, hours away from home. Two days later, my blood pressure went extremely high and William's heart rate went extremely low, so I had an emergency C-section. This turned out to be a blessing because attempting a vaginal delivery would have likely resulted in complications for both William and me due to William's immediately evident craniosynostosis; his skull would not have been able to mold appropriately to fit through the birth canal. It was also a blessing that I had to be transferred to the hospital with the NICU with so many specialists available.

Due to my own health condition with the HELLP syndrome, I was not able to be awake for the C-section, as I had to have general anesthesia. Everything I know about the first day of William's life is from what others have told me; I was in rough shape and don't remember anything about the day of or day after the delivery. My mom and William's father were present for the delivery, and my mom told me later that she asked about his head shape right away as it was quite evident right at birth. William's Apgar score* was only 2, and he struggled to breathe right after he was born. The specialists attempted to put in a breathing tube to help him, but it was apparent right away that his anatomy was a bit different, as the breathing tube would not go in. An emergency ultrasound revealed that he had a condition known as esophageal atresia, meaning his esophagus, which is what carries the food from the mouth to the stomach, doesn't completely attach to the stomach.

Fortunately, William was soon able to breathe on his own and he stabilized in the hours after delivery. He was placed in the NICU with many IV and other monitoring lines attached to him and additional tests being performed in those first days. I met William the day after he was born while he was in the NICU. His father and I attended morning rounds, where the different specialists met to discuss the plan. We learned then that fixing the esophageal atresia was priority one so that William would be able to eat. This surgery was done within three days of his birth and it went well. Even so, he still had some issues with feeding and swallowing due to the constriction in his esophagus and scar tissue from the surgery, so we had to use a device known as a nipple shield to help slow the flow of his feeding.

---

* The Apgar score is an evaluation used right after birth (at one minute and five minutes) to assess the newborn's health (heart rate, muscle tone, and other signs) using a scale of 0 to 10, with the higher score indicating more reassuring signs.[228]

Discussions next turned to the shape of his head, which looked like a cloverleaf, with bulging at the sides. We were told he had severe bicoronal craniosynostosis, but that it didn't need to be fixed right away, so after about 30 days in the NICU, William was able to go home with us. We knew that we would be returning later to have genetic testing done, as the doctors were fairly confident William had syndromic CS.

It was great to be home, but we did have a few scares. At one point it was recommended that we stop using the nipple shield for feeding. However, William was not able to handle that and started choking and turned blue with a feeding. I had to perform CPR and call 911. Thankfully, William was fine. Some feeding issues continued as he grew, and he was supported with feeding therapy until about age three.

He also had a seizure as an infant and needed to spend some time back in the hospital to be evaluated. Thankfully, he was able to be weaned off anti-seizure medicine after he was about one year old.

When William was three months old, the genetic testing revealed that the type of craniosynostosis William has is Muenke syndrome, which we had never heard of before. Neither my nor his father's family had any known history of this syndrome. The genetics appointment was a lot to take in, and we didn't feel great after it.

We met with the craniofacial team and planned for the open surgical repair to correct William's skull shape, which he had at five months of age. William also needed a second surgery since he had hydrocephalus and a Chiari malformation.

William had to go through extensive occupational therapy and physical therapy. His head was so heavy and disproportionate that he couldn't sit by himself, and he needed lots of strengthening of his neck and core. He also eventually needed some speech therapy, but he has now graduated out of that. He still gets some physical therapy and occupational therapy to this day.

William saw the ophthalmologist early on and got his first pair of glasses at 10 months old. He has done eyepatch therapy since six months of age and needed eye surgery for strabismus (misaligned eyes) when he was five. He recently had a follow-up with eye specialists that show his eyes are improving; we just got the all clear to not come back to see them for an entire year!

William does have some ongoing issues in his mouth such as a high-arched palate, adult teeth that are struggling to come through, and some overcrowding. He may need a palate expander at some point to help create extra space for his teeth to come in. He has always struggled with opening his mouth wide. He has also suffered from sleep disruptions and night terrors since he was little. His tonsils are slightly enlarged and being monitored.

He continues to get hearing tests as we have been told that hearing loss may occur as he enters adulthood; so far, his hearing is good.

We had originally planned to homeschool William, but then decided to put him in kindergarten at age six. It was a tough transition for him, but his intellectual level has always been on par with his classmates, and he has never needed additional help with reading or math. He actually really enjoys math!

Today, William is eight years old in second grade. He has a younger sister, who is five, who has never shown any signs of Muenke syndrome. Just like any other active eight year old, William enjoys playing outside. He tried soccer but seems to enjoy individual activities more such as playing with Lego or Magna-Tiles, and he is extremely curious about how everything works.

Going through this journey with William has been incredibly hard, yet beautiful at the same time. To witness your child literally transform before your eyes is indescribable. We are so blessed to have amazing doctors and surgeons!

Being a first-time parent was scary enough, but adding in an emergency birth, myriad health complications, and test results that I couldn't understand felt like a punch to the gut and an impossible mountain to climb. I'm so grateful for the people from our town and from the cranio community who came alongside me and our family. Going to Keegan's 5K for Craniosynostosis Awareness (Comstock 2023) each summer is always a highlight for us!

My faith has been tested many times, and yet there were moments even in the scariest situations where I had a peace that I couldn't explain, but I just knew William would be okay. William has been so strong and so brave since the minute he was born. I'm so incredibly blessed to be his mom and to support him as he continues to conquer the battles he faces. He has overcome so much in just eight years of life. He is my hero! I hope and pray that any other parents on this journey can feel the same support from this book, the cranio community that continues to grow, and from the friends and family around them.

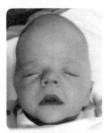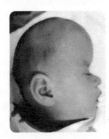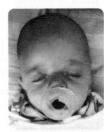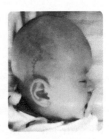

William, before his CS repair surgery at five months of age (left two photos) and after (right two photos).

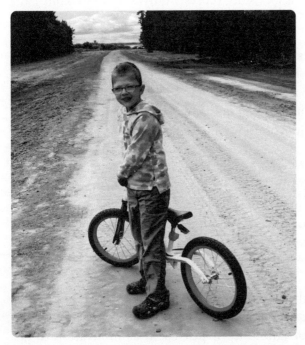

William, present day, enjoying a bike ride on a family vacation.

Michael, an adult, from Minnesota, US, living with Apert syndrome

Living with Apert syndrome isn't always easy. I'm 18 years old, and I've had 33 surgeries so far.

Hospital stays after surgeries are not very fun. The IVs (intravenous lines) are always annoying with the very sticky tape, the nurses come in what feels like every two minutes to check your vital signs, and if you stay for more than a few days, it messes with your regular sleep schedule for the next month. However, if it wasn't for those surgeries, I wouldn't be the person I am today.

There are a few bright sides to having medical differences too. For example, in 2014, I was invited along with one kid from every state on a special trip to Orlando, Florida, and Washington, D.C., where I got to tour the White House and meet the "First Dogs" (the US presidents' pet dogs) at the time, as well as Michelle Obama. I've also had the opportunity to advocate for other kids and people with special needs by talking to local and Minnesota state representatives, both in Saint Paul and Washington D.C.

I've met various athletes through the years, at events either sponsored or hosted by Gillette Children's. Through Gillette's partnership with the Minnesota Twins [baseball team], I even had the opportunity once to throw out the first pitch at a game, and I've met a good number of players thanks to the opportunities Gillette has provided.

Most importantly, the doctors I've had over the years have been really kind, and they have helped me be who I am today. I can do most "normal" things in life, but due to my syndrome, I have limited hand and shoulder mobility, which seems to be the main difference that remains, even after all my surgeries. After certain surgeries, I felt insecure about doing certain movements, but I've learned to adapt to the way my body works.

When I was younger, other kids would either stare or make fun of me, and I would feel a little sad. But as I've grown older, I've learned to give a wave and say, "Hi" or ignore it, or just use it as motivation to get stronger. It doesn't bother me as much anymore.

Starting in middle school, I joined band and played the trumpet. I enjoyed it and continued playing in high school where it was so much more fun. High school was a lot of fun, even during the COVID year, and I made many friends and memories in the band. I was told by my craniofacial surgeon and orthodontist that not many people with craniofacial syndromes can play an instrument, so I was fortunate and lucky that I succeeded with the trumpet.

Apert syndrome certainly has presented challenges, but after 18 years of living with it, I don't really feel that much different than other people, and it's even given me some great opportunities that I would not have experienced without it.

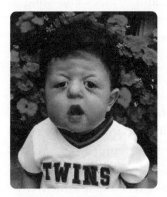 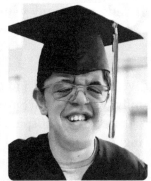 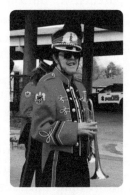

Left to right: Michael, at 10 months of age; age 18, at his high school graduation; age 18, in the band.

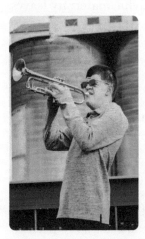 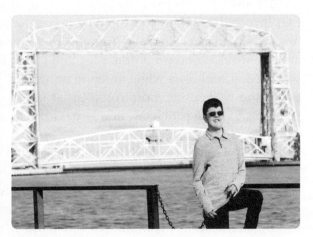

Michael, age 18, playing the trumpet (left) and enjoying the outdoors (right).

Sarah, mother of six-year-old Emily, from Minnesota, US

I always knew that I wanted to have children, but I kind of secretly (or maybe not so secretly), wanted to have a girl. I always dreamed of baking cupcakes and watching *Beauty and the Beast* with my daughter. When my husband, Alex, and I found out we were pregnant, I tried not to get my hopes up. Then, just like that, we were at our 20-week appointment hearing the news that it was a girl. We were thrilled.

As the pregnancy progressed, we did our best to prepare for the changes that having a child would bring to our lives. Like a lot of other first-time parents, we did our research. We read books and articles and sought out the advice of our friends and family who already had kids. As the due date grew nearer, we felt like we were as ready as we could possibly hope to be.

I went into labor on a Wednesday night and endured a tough few days before our daughter, Emily, was born on Saturday morning. We hadn't slept at all since Wednesday, and the hospital had no nursery. She cried in our room the entire night despite our desperate attempts to make her comfortable. We quickly realized we had no idea what we were getting into. I think part of that is unavoidable, but I also feel like it's due to the way we often romanticize the experience of having a child.

I had heard accounts from my coworkers about idyllic maternity leaves that involved cuddling and catching up on Netflix. This was certainly not my experience. Those first few weeks, Emily had trouble sleeping and she wouldn't take a bottle. Alex and I were both so tired and overwhelmed, it took us a while to figure things out. Eventually, things got easier and we became more confident as parents, but even as you find solutions to some problems, new issues arise to take their place.

At Emily's two-month checkup, our pediatrician noticed she was developing a flat spot on one side of the back of her head. It took me by total surprise. Once it was pointed out, it was obvious, and I started to look for every opportunity to keep her off that side of her head—including shifting her head in the middle of the night. If you have ever tried to move the head of a sleeping baby without waking them, you know it's treacherous stuff. We did the best we could, but when we arrived at her four-month doctor's visit, we could see it wasn't getting any better. We were given the choice to take her to a specialist or to just watch and see; the pediatrician did not think it was that severe and said that as her hair grew, we would probably not notice it.

Fortunately, at the time, I was working at Gillette Children's. I knew they had the expertise to evaluate and treat my daughter. We decided we wanted to have her evaluated and, without hesitation, this is where we chose to bring her. After a visit with a craniofacial surgeon to assess Emily's head shape, we were told she had deformational plagiocephaly. The next step would be getting her fitted for a helmet orthosis.

The process went smoothly. First, they took a 3D scan of Emily's head, then created an exact model of it with a 3D printer. The helmet orthosis was then molded around the model.

It took a couple of weeks before we could return to pick up the helmet, and after that we went in for a fitting where a few adjustments were made. We got our instructions, and voilà! Emily had her newest accessory. I made sure to add a couple bows to doll it up a bit since she would be wearing it for 23 hours a day for the next several months.

As a new parent, there's a lot that you worry about. I worried about the effect the helmet would have on Emily. Would she be uncomfortable? Would the helmet be hot to wear, especially during the summer? Would she still sleep, or would her sleep schedule be disrupted?

Emily did well with her helmet, with just one minor issue. About a week into wearing it, she got a small scratch on the side of her face from the cap rubbing her cheek. We had to take her back in to get the area checked and have her helmet adjusted. After that, she wore her helmet like a champ. Sure, she got sweaty sometimes, and at other times it felt inconvenient, but the months just flew by. In the end, we were happy with our decision to have her fit for a helmet and wouldn't change it for the world.

Emily is now a thriving six-year-old who prefers wearing bows to helmets. She thinks it's funny when we tell her about her little helmet, and we even kept it to show it to her. Her biggest concern when she looks at the helmet today was how her head was ever that small.

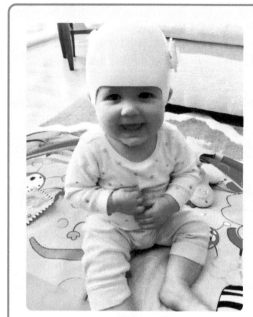

Emily, wearing her helmet.

Chapter 9

Further reading and research

Education is not the filling of a pail,
but the lighting of a fire.
William Butler Yeats

Further reading

For those who would like further reading on this condition, a list of rec-ommended books, websites, and resources has been collated and will be regularly updated. Access to the list is provided in **Useful web resources.**

Research

Research serves as a cornerstone of evidence-based medicine and drives health care advancement. We discussed the importance of evidence-based medicine (or evidence-based practice) in Chapter 1. It is "the conscientious, explicit, and judicious use of current best evidence in making decisions about the care of individual patients." It combines the best available external clinical evidence from research with the clinical expertise of the professional.[70] Family priorities and preferences are also considered.[229]

Evidence is collected by carrying out scientific studies (research studies), the results of which are published as full-length, peer-reviewed research articles (or papers) in scientific journals. "Peer-reviewed" means that experts with relevant content knowledge have reviewed, challenged, and agreed that the scientific method and study conclusions based on the results are sound.

Scientific studies may also be presented in brief at conferences, and conference proceedings are often published. However, conference proceedings present preliminary results and peer review is minimal. *Therefore, full-length published research articles are the most rigorous and sound evidence.*

The above published research outputs are collectively known as scientific literature or, simply, research.

Research may also be discussed on various social media platforms such as X (formerly Twitter), Facebook, LinkedIn, and Instagram. If you consume information this way, it is always important to go back to the original source (i.e., the full-length research article) to ensure the media's portrayal of the study findings is accurate.

You may have familiarity with searching the scientific literature. If not, search engines such as PubMed (ncbi.nlm.nih.gov/pubmed) and Google Scholar (scholar.google.com) are good places to start. They provide a free abstract (a short summary of the article), which can be very useful. In the past, you generally needed to belong to an academic or medical institution to have access to full-length research articles. Many articles are now available online for free. Google Scholar provides links to many full-length articles, and some community libraries allow you to request full-length articles.

You might have heard the phrase, "Just because someone says it doesn't mean it's true." This is worth remembering in all aspects of life, but it is also relevant to research. While research articles go through a peer review process, you should still read them with a critical eye. Ask yourself, How confident can I be in the results of this research study? Was the sample size big enough to be representative of the larger population? Did the results support the conclusion?

If you aren't a trained scientist, reviewing the quality of the evidence might be more challenging, but you can still make sure the basic methods make sense and the author's conclusions are supported by the data presented. The information below will help you learn about some research study designs and how study design affects how much confidence you can place in a study's conclusions.

Research study design

There are different research study designs, and each has its value. The quality of the evidence, or level of evidence, is graded based on the study design and how well the methods were executed. Research articles sometimes list (often in the abstract) the level of evidence from I to V, with level I being the highest.

The most common research study designs, listed from highest to lowest level of evidence, are:

- Systematic review
- Randomized controlled trial
- Cohort
- Case control
- Cross-sectional
- Case report and case series

Systematic review: A systematic review summarizes the results of several scientific studies on the same topic. They can be qualitative (descriptive) or quantitative (numerical):

- Qualitative: A summary of common themes and findings across studies but without a statistical analysis.
- Quantitative: A statistical analysis carried out that takes a weighted average of the findings across studies to produce one estimate for the effect of a treatment, for example. The quantitative approach is called a "meta-analysis."

The highest level of evidence is a systematic review of randomized controlled trials (described next), although systematic reviews can also include studies that used other types of study designs. Systematic reviews may be published by individual researchers or groups. The Cochrane collaboration is a worldwide association of researchers, health care professionals, patients, and carers that publishes systematic reviews on various topics.

Randomized controlled trial (RCT): An RCT is a study design aimed at identifying cause and effect. The cause is, for example, the treatment, and the effect is the outcome being measured. Strict control of the study method (the "C" in RCT) helps to ensure the treatment of interest is the only factor that could cause the outcome. A treatment group receives the treatment while a nontreatment group (also known as the control group) does not. The participants are randomly assigned (the "R" in RCT) to one of the groups. The random assignment is one of the key strengths of this study design because it takes care of the "unknown unknowns" that may influence the outcome. The treatment effect is found by comparing the outcomes of the treatment and nontreatment groups. RCTs are considered the highest quality study design but are still uncommon in medical literature.

Cohort: A cohort is a group of people who share a common characteristic (e.g., diagnosis, gender). In a cohort study, outcome is measured two or more times. Researchers identify the characteristic of interest and then measure the outcome, looking for associations between the two. A cohort study is a form of longitudinal study ("longitudinal" means that the same outcome is measured on the same participants two or more times over a period of time). You may come across the terms "prospective" and "retrospective" cohort studies.

- In prospective cohort studies, research questions and methods are defined, and a cohort is followed over time, collecting data.
- In retrospective cohort studies, research questions and methods are defined after data has been collected or already exists (e.g., a person's medical record).

Case control: In case control studies, researchers identify the outcome of interest, which defines the groups (e.g., infants with a specific diagnosis and typically developing infants), and then look backward in time at different factors or exposures that might have caused different outcomes. At the beginning of the study, the outcome is known, but the factors or exposures that might have caused that outcome are unknown. This is the opposite of cohort studies. Because the outcome and factors or exposures data already exist, case control studies are always retrospective.

Cross-sectional: Cross-sectional studies take measurements only once from participants. Researchers look for associations between certain factors and exposures, and outcomes.

Case report and case series: A case report (also referred to as a single-subject case study) is an account of a single patient—usually a unique case—and their medical history, status, and outcomes from a treatment, for example. A case series is a group of case reports on patients who were exposed to a similar treatment. These reports are usually retrospective, and data has already been collected by other means (usually as part of routine medical care).

Getting involved in research

There are many opportunities to become involved in research. Together with medical professionals and researchers, people with lived experience can help drive advancement in health care.

a) As a participant

Researchers working in academic and medical settings are always looking for participants for their studies. You might receive an invitation to participate in such a study via an email, letter in the mail, phone call, social media ad, or other method.

Some studies are very easy and may just involve completing one online survey; others may take more time with various measurements being taken on more than one occasion. Just as you are advised to read published research studies with a critical eye, so should you judge new research study opportunities before agreeing to participate. Participating can take time and effort—the expected time commitment will be communicated in the study recruitment material. There is often a small reimbursement offered for time spent in a study.

It's worth noting that you, as the study participant, may not personally benefit from the research study, but the collective population with the condition will likely benefit.

Clinical trials are research studies conducted to evaluate the safety and effectiveness of new medical treatments, including new medications and devices before they can be approved for widespread use. They are often conducted following a randomized controlled trial research study design.

A potential benefit of participating in clinical trials is gaining early access to new medical treatments. Even if you are assigned to the control group (which usually receives standard care), you may have early access to the new treatment once the data collection phase is complete. In addition, standard care is likely to be current best practice.

You can find information about clinical trials through various sources:

- The National Institutes of Health in the US maintains a comprehensive database, ClinicalTrials.gov, where you can learn about clinical trials around the world. You can search this database by specific medical condition, location, or other pertinent criteria to identify relevant clinical trials that may be currently enrolling participants.
- Major academic medical centers, research institutions, and hospitals often conduct clinical trials and can provide information about their ongoing studies.
- Medical professionals may be aware of ongoing clinical trials in their field and can provide guidance to families who are interested in participating.
- Organizations that support particular conditions are another source of information.

Depending on the nature of the treatment in the clinical trial, you may want to, or be required to, consult with your medical professional to help you consider the risks and benefits of participating.

b) As a co-producer

Family engagement in research (FER) plays a crucial role in fostering collaboration and helping improve study design and outcome. When families become involved in research as collaborators on a study rather than simply as participants, researchers gain valuable insights into the lived experiences and perspectives of families. Families participate at every stage of the research process: concept, design, planning, conduct, and reporting of the study findings. These opportunities are still rare but are becoming more common. As an example, a link to the FER program at Gillette Children's is included in **Useful web resources.**

The family engagement in research movement is largely attributed to the similar and earlier patient and public involvement initiative in the UK. Here are some opportunities:

- **CanChild** and the **Kids Brain Health Network** in Canada currently offer The Family Engagement in Research program, a short online training course through McMaster University Continuing Education to train family members and researchers (including coordinators and assistants) in collaborating on research.

- Online training modules are available at **Patient-Oriented Research Curriculum in Child Health (PORCCH)**.
- The **Patient-Centered Outcomes Research Institute (PCORI)** and the **Strategy for Patient-Oriented Research (SPOR)** are two other organizations that encourage family engagement.

USEFUL WEB RESOURCES

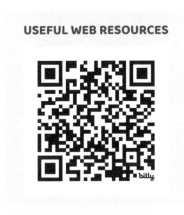

Acknowledgments

It takes a village to raise a child
African proverb

And it takes a village to produce a Healthcare Series. Publication of this series began with an idea, then with five titles, and then more titles. These acknowledgments relate to the entire series.

The formula of deep medical information interspersed with lived experience gives readers an appreciation of the childhood-acquired, often lifelong conditions. We thank the many people who contributed to each title: medical professionals at Gillette Children's who willingly came forward to lead each book; Gillette writers who did the research and writing of each; other Gillette team members who contributed from their different specialties; family authors and vignette writers who shared their personal stories; other families who shared photographs; the Gillette editing team who ensured the content and structure worked for the reader; Olwyn Roche who beautifully illustrated each title; advance readers, both professionals and families, whose feedback was invaluable; and Lina Abdennabi who coordinated Gillette Press operations. Behind every book was also a pit team who converted the finished manuscript into the book you now hold. Ruth Wilson led and looked after copyediting and proofreading. Jazmin Welch created the beautiful design and layout. Audrey McClellan indexed each title.

Smoothly creating each title required great teamwork among our villagers.

Staff at Gillette Children's provided continual support to the project and everyone involved. This included the steering committee, in particular Paula Montgomery, Dr. Micah Niermann, and Barbara Joers.

This Healthcare Series is co-published with Mac Keith Press. From the get-go, the journey with Ann-Marie Halligan and Sally Wilkinson was one of great support and collaboration.

Gillette Children's Healthcare Press

Glossary

TERM	DEFINITION
Abnormal/atypical	Deviating from the typical expectation.
Adenotonsillar hypertrophy	Enlarged tonsils and adenoids.
Anesthesiologist	A medical professional who specializes in the evaluation, care, and monitoring during, before, and after surgery while delivering anesthesia.
Ankylosis	Immobility and fusion of a joint; leads to stiffness and rigidity in the joint.
Anterior	Near the front, or front side.
Anterior plagiocephaly	A skewed head shape in which the head is flat on one side typically seen with unicoronal craniosynostosis.
Aortic coarctation	A narrowing of the main vessel in the heart.
Assisted ventilation	The use of an external device to help a person breathe; may be invasive or noninvasive.
Brachycephaly	A short and wide head shape typically seen with bicoronal craniosynostosis.
Brachydactyly	A condition in which fingers and toes are shorter than typical.
Broadening	Becoming larger in distance from side to side; widening.
Cerebrospinal fluid leak	A leak of fluid that surrounds the brain and spinal canal.
Chiari malformation	A condition in which the brain tissue extends into the spinal canal instead of staying within the skull.
Cleft palate	An opening or split in the roof of the mouth.

Clinodactyly	A condition in which fingers are bent or curved.
Congenital	Referring to a condition that is present from birth.
Congenital muscular torticollis (CMT)	The persistent shortening of one of the sternocleidomastoid muscles. When described as "congenital," it means this condition is present from birth.
Corneal damage	Damage to the cornea, a transparent layer on the front surface of the eye, which may cause vision impairment or loss.
Cranial	Relating to the skull.
Cranial (cephalic) index (CI)	The maximum width of the skull divided by the maximum length of the skull; expressed as a percentage.
Cranial vault	The space that encases and protects the brain.
Deformational plagiocephaly	An abnormal head shape that develops from external pressure on the skull bones, typically from positioning; also called "positional" or "occipital" plagiocephaly.
Deformity	A malformed or misshapen part of the body.
De novo	A Latin term meaning "from the beginning," "new"; a *de novo* gene mutation occurs for the first time in a child, but not in either parent.
Dental crowding	The overlapping or misalignment of teeth.
Ectopic teeth	Teeth outside the typical position.
Embryo	A developing human from conception up to the end of the eighth week after conception.
Endoscopic approach	A procedure using special instruments that allow the surgeon to work through small incisions.
Epicanthal fold	A skinfold of the upper eyelid that covers the inner corner of the eye.
Epilepsy	A neurological disorder in which brain activity becomes abnormal, causing seizures or periods of unusual behavior, sensations, and sometimes loss of awareness. See *seizure*.

Eruption of teeth	The process of teeth pushing through the gums into the mouth.
Fetus	A developing human from the eighth week after conception to birth.
Fontanel	An open spot (often called a "soft spot") in an infant's skull where the corners of the skull bones meet. Fontanels occur at the junction of the sutures and most close within the first two years of life. See *suture*.
Fusion	The process of joining two or more things together to form one.
Gastrostomy tube (G-tube)	A device that is surgically inserted into the stomach; can be used to deliver nutrition; also called a PEG tube.
Gene	The basic unit of heredity that is transferred from parent to offspring.
Genetic	Referring to genes or heredity.
Health-related quality of life (HRQOL)	The way in which a condition affects a person's well-being.
Helical folds	Folds of the external ear.
High-arched palate	A narrow, tall roof of the mouth. See *palate*.
Hydrocephalus	A condition in which there is a buildup of cerebrospinal fluid in cavities (ventricles) in the brain.
Hypertelorism	Spacing between the eyes that is wider than typical.
Hypotelorism	Spacing between the eyes that is narrower than typical.
Infant	A child from birth to one year of age.
Intracranial pressure (ICP)	The measure of pressure inside the skull.
Jejunostomy tube (J-tube)	A device inserted into a section of the small intestine; can be used to deliver nutrition.
Lateral	Away from the midline (or middle of the body), referring to the side.
Maxillary hypoplasia	Underdevelopment of the upper jaw.

Midface hypoplasia	Underdevelopment of the middle of the face, causing the upper jaw, cheekbones, and eye sockets to appear sunken.
Morbidity rate	The measure of the number of temporary or permanent disabilities that occur due to a specific illness or condition.
Mortality rate	The measure of the number of deaths that occur due to a specific illness or condition.
Multidisciplinary	Coordinated treatment by medical professionals from a number of disciplines.
Multisuture CS	Craniosynostosis that involves the premature fusion of more than one suture. See *suture*.
Nasal root deviation	Atypical alignment of the top of the nose where the nasal bones meet the frontal bones; the nose deviates toward the fused suture.
Nasogastric tube (NG tube)	A device inserted through the nose and into the stomach; can be used to deliver nutrition.
Nasolacrimal duct stenosis	Blocked or narrowed (stenosis) eye duct; a condition of the eyes that causes decreased tear production and may lead to increased eye infections.
Nasopharyngeal airway device	A device inserted into the nose to create an open path for airflow when the airway space is constricted.
Neuropsychological testing	Individualized assessment of the skills and abilities linked to coordinated brain function, such as memory, cognition, perception, problem-solving, and verbal abilities and how they relate to behavior.
Newborn	A child from birth to four weeks.
Noninvasive ventilation	A type of assisted ventilation that delivers pressure into the lungs using a device such as a CPAP (continuous positive airway pressure) machine or a BiPAP (bilevel positive airway pressure) machine. "Noninvasive" refers to the method used to administer the ventilation through the nose or mouth, rather than directly into the airway, as occurs with invasive ventilation. See *assistive ventilation*.
Nonsyndromic	An isolated condition, not part of a syndrome.

Normocephaly	Normal head structure.
Nurse practitioner	A registered nurse with advanced training, able to provide assessment, diagnosis, and treatment along with preventive health maintenance.
Obstructive sleep apnea	A disorder in which a person frequently stops breathing during their sleep.
Occipital	Referring to being situated in the back of the head; the back of the head or skull.
Ophthalmologist	A medical professional who specializes in the care of the eyes.
Orthodontist	A medical professional who specializes in the care of teeth and jaw alignment.
Orthosis	A device designed to hold specific body parts in position to modify their structure and/or function; also called a brace.
Ossification	The process of turning material into bone.
Otitis media	An inflammation of the middle ear. Otitis media with effusion is a collection of fluid in the middle ear in the absence of an ear infection.
Otolaryngologist	A medical professional who specializes in the care of the ears, nose, and throat.
Palate	The roof of the mouth; it separates the mouth from the nasal cavity.
Papilledema	A swelling of the optic nerve in the eye due to increased intracranial pressure. See *intracranial pressure*.
Patent ductus arteriosus	A condition in which a hole is present in the main vessel of the heart at birth.
Pathologic	Referring to the involvement, cause, or nature of a condition.
Peritoneal cavity	A space in the abdominal area, not occupied by abdominal organs; used as an emptying space for a VP shunt. See *ventriculoperitoneal shunt*.

Physician assistant	A medical professional licensed to practice medicine in every specialty and setting in the United States and other jurisdictions. Physician assistants require graduate schooling, have greater medical privileges than nurses, and work alongside a supervising physician.
Posterior	Near the back, or back side.
Posterior plagiocephaly	A skewed head shape in which the head is flat on one side or on the back of the head typically seen with lambdoid craniosynostosis or deformational plagiocephaly.
Premature	Referring to something occurring too early or before the usual or proper time.
Prevalence	The proportion of the population who have a particular disease or attribute at a specified point in time or over a specified period of time.
Proptosis	A condition in which the eyes appear to be bulging; also called "exorbitism" or "exophthalmos."
Ptosis	A condition of one or both of the upper eyelids drooping over the eye.
Risk factor	An aspect of personal behavior or lifestyle, an environmental exposure, or a hereditary characteristic that is associated with an increase in the occurrence of a particular disease, injury, or other health condition.
Scaphocephaly	A classification of CS characterized by a boat-shaped head typically seen with sagittal craniosynostosis.
Sedation	The administration of medications to produce a state of calm or sleep.
Seizure	A sudden, uncontrolled, abnormal burst of electrical activity in the brain that may cause changes in the level of consciousness, behavior, memory, or feelings.
Sensorineural hearing loss	Hearing loss that occurs due to damage to the inner ear, impacting low frequency (deep, low-pitched) sounds the most.
Septum	The partition between the nostrils.

Single suture CS	Craniosynostosis that involves the premature fusion of one suture. See *fusion*.
Strabismus	Atypical alignment of the eyes, often appearing as crossed eyes.
Stroke	A condition when a blood vessel in the brain is either blocked or ruptured.
Superior	Situated above; looking down from above.
Supraorbital rim	The bony ridge above the eye sockets; makes up the brow bone, located at the bottom edge of the frontal bone
Suture	The immovable junction between two bones; cranial sutures are fibrous joints that connect the bones of the skull. (Not to be confused with stitches, which are also called sutures.)
Symphalangism	Stiffness of joints due to ankylosis. See *ankylosis*.
Syndactyly	The union of two or more fingers or toes, also termed "webbing"; may include bony fusion of adjacent digits. When the union is incomplete (digits are not fully conjoined or joined only by skin instead of bone), it is referred to as partial syndactyly. See *fusion*.
Syndrome	A group of characteristics and findings that consistently occur together and indicate a specific condition.
Syndromic	Referring to a characteristic that occurs as part of a syndrome.
Synostosis	The union or fusion of two or more separate bones to form a single bone. See *fusion*.
Tracheal cartilaginous sleeve (TCS)	A malformation where the typical rings of cartilage in the trachea are replaced with a sleeve of cartilage.
Tracheostomy	A medical procedure that involves creating an opening in the neck and placing a tube in the trachea to allow the passage of air.
Trigonocephaly	A classification of CS characterized by a triangular-shaped head typically seen with metopic craniosynostosis.

Tube Feeding	A method of delivering liquid nutrition though a plastic tube that has been placed in the stomach or small intestine.
Turribrachycephaly	A classification of CS characterized by a tower or cone-shaped head with flat, prominent, elongated forehead and temporal widening on both sides along with occipital flattening typically seen with various forms of syndromic craniosynostosis.
Ventriculomegaly	A condition characterized by enlarged ventricles in the brain.
Ventriculoperitoneal shunt (VP shunt)	A device inserted into the ventricles of the brain; the shunt tubing (catheter) drains the cerebrospinal fluid from the ventricles and transports it to a reservoir where it is stored and then pumped to the peritoneal cavity (a space within the abdominal area not occupied by the abdominal organs). There, the fluid is absorbed by the body.
Vertebrae	The bones that form the spine.

References

1. World Health Organization (2001) *International classification of functioning, disability and health (ICF)*. [online] Available at: <https://www.who.int/standards/classifications/international-classification-of-functioning-disability-and-health> [Accessed February 22 2024].

2. Kajdic N, Spazzapan P, Velnar T (2018) Craniosynostosis - recognition, clinical characteristics, and treatment. *Bosn J Basic Med Sci*, 18, 110-116.

3. Dempsey RF, Monson LA, Maricevich RS, et al. (2019) Nonsyndromic craniosynostosis. *Clin Plast Surg*, 46, 123-139.

4. Bautista G (2021) Craniosynostosis: Neonatal perspectives. *Neoreviews*, 22, 250-257.

5. Forrest CR, Nguyen PD, Smith DM (2017) Craniosynostosis. In: Bentz M, editor, *Principles & practice of pediatric plastic surgery*. Boca Raton: CRC Press, pp 595-647.

6. Persing JA, Jane JA, Shaffrey M (1989) Virchow and the pathogenesis of craniosynostosis: A translation of his original work. *Plast Reconstr Surg*, 83, 738-42.

7. Dias MS, Samson T, Rizk EB, et al. (2020) Identifying the misshapen head: Craniosynostosis and related disorders. *Pediatrics*, 146, 1-20.

8. Andersson H, Gomes SP (1968) Craniosynostosis. Review of the literature and indications for surgery. *Acta Paediatr Scand*, 57, 47-54.

9. American Trauma Society (2024) *Trauma center levels explained*. [online] Available at: <https://www.amtrauma.org/page/traumalevels> [Accessed January 19 2024].

10. American Academy of Physician Associates (2024) *What is a PA?* [online] Available at: <https://www.aapa.org/about/what-is-a-pa/> [Accessed January 19 2024].

11. American Academy of Pediatrics (2023) Recommendations for preventive pediatric health care. [pdf] Illinois, American Academy of Pediatrics, Available at: <https://downloads.aap.org/AAP/PDF/periodicity_schedule.pdf?_ga=2.189158946.881015920.1689013444-1582860731.1673531157> [Accessed April 24 2024].

12. Jin SW, Sim KB, Kim SD (2016) Development and growth of the normal cranial vault: An embryologic review. *J Korean Neurosurg Soc*, 59, 192-6.

13. Merriam Webster (2024a) *Prenatal*. [online] Available at: <https://www.merriam-webster.com/dictionary/prenatal> [Accessed March 28 2024].

14. Merriam Webster (2024b) *Perinatal*. [online] Available at: <https://www.merriam-webster.com/dictionary/perinatal> [Accessed January 19 2024].

15. Flaherty K, Singh N, Richtsmeier JT (2016) Understanding craniosynostosis as a growth disorder. *Wiley Interdiscip Rev Dev Biol*, 5, 429-59.

16. Mathijssen IM, Van Splunder J, Vermeij-Keers C, et al. (1999) Tracing cranio-synostosis to its developmental stage through bone center displacement. *J Craniofac Genet Dev Biol*, 19, 57-63.

17. Centers for Disease Control and Prevention (2021) *Infants (0-1 year of age).* [online] Available at: <https://www.cdc.gov/ncbddd/childdevelopment/positive parenting/infants.html> [Accessed January 19 2024].

18. Proctor MR, Meara JG (2019) A review of the management of single-suture craniosynostosis, past, present, and future. *J Neurosurg Pediatr*, 24, 622-631.

19. Vu GH, Xu W, Go BC, et al. (2021) Physiologic timeline of cranial-base suture and synchondrosis closure. *Plast Reconstr Surg*, 148, 973-982.

20. Marbate T, Kedia S, Gupta DK (2022) Evaluation and management of nonsyn-dromic craniosynostosis. *J Pediatr Neurosci*, 17, 77-91.

21. Ruengdit S, Troy Case D, Mahakkanukrauh P (2020) Cranial suture closure as an age indicator: A review. *Forensic Sci Int*, 307, 1-11.

22. Hersh DS, Bookland MJ, Hughes CD (2021) Diagnosis and management of suture-related concerns of the infant skull. *Pediatr Clin North Am*, 68, 727-742.

23. Lipsett B, Reddy V, Steanson K (2023) *Anatomy, head and neck: Fontanelles.* [e-book] Treasure Island (FL), StatPearls Publishing. Available at: National Library of Medicine <https://www.ncbi.nlm.nih.gov/books/NBK542197/> [Accessed March 29 2024].

24. Yapijakis C, Pachis N, Sotiriadou T, et al. (2023) Molecular mechanisms involved in craniosynostosis. *In Vivo*, 37, 36-46.

25. National Human Genome Research Institute (2024) *Syndrome.* [online] Available at: <https://www.genome.gov/genetics-glossary/Syndrome> [Accessed January 19 2024].

26. Blessing M, Gallagher ER (2022) Epidemiology, genetics, and pathophysiology of craniosynostosis. *Oral Maxillofac Surg Clin North Am*, 34, 341-352.

27. Jha RT, Magge SN, Keating RF (2018) Diagnosis and surgical options for cranio-synostosis. In: Ellenbogen R, Sekhar, L, Kitchen, N, editors, *Principles of neurological surgery*. Amsterdam: Elsevier, pp 148-169.

28. Betances EM, Mendez MD, Das JM (2023) *Craniosynostosis.* [e-book] Treasure Island (FL), StatPearls Publishing. Available at: National Library of Medicine <https://www.ncbi.nlm.nih.gov/books/NBK544366/#_NBK544366_pubdet_> [Accessed February 24 2024].

29. Centers for Disease Control and Prevention (2023) *Prevalence.* [online] Available at: <https://www.cdc.gov/nchs/hus/sources-definitions/prevalence.htm> [Accessed January 19 2024].

30. Shlobin NA, Baticulon RE, Ortega CA, et al. (2022) Global epidemiology of craniosynostosis: A systematic review and meta-analysis. *World Neurosurg*, 164, 413-423.

31. Cornelissen M, Ottelander B, Rizopoulos D, et al. (2016) Increase of prevalence of craniosynostosis. *J Craniomaxillofac Surg*, 44, 1273-9.

32. Schraw JM, Woodhouse JP, Langlois PH, et al. (2021) Risk factors and time trends for isolated craniosynostosis. *Birth Defects Res*, 113, 43-54.

33. Lee HQ, Hutson JM, Wray AC, et al. (2012) Changing epidemiology of nonsyn-dromic craniosynostosis and revisiting the risk factors. *Journal of Craniofacial Surgery,* 23, 1245-1251.

34. Centers for Disease Control and Prevention (2015) *Epidemiology glossary.* [online] Available at: <https://www.cdc.gov/reproductivehealth/data_stats/glossary .html> [Accessed January 19 2024].

35. Sacks GN, Skolnick GB, Trachtenberg A, et al. (2019) The impact of ethnicity on craniosynostosis in the United States. *J Craniofac Surg,* 30, 2526-2529.

36. Anderson IA, Goomany A, Bonthron DT, et al. (2014) Does patient ethnicity affect site of craniosynostosis? *J Neurosurg Pediatr,* 14, 682-7.

37. Greenwood J, Flodman P, Osann K, Boyadjiev SA, Kimonis V (2014) Familial incidence and associated symptoms in a population of individuals with nonsyn-dromic craniosynostosis. *Genet Med,* 16, 302-10.

38. Abdelhamid K, Konci R, Elhawary H, Gorgy A, Smith L (2021) Advanced parental age: Is it contributing to an increased incidence of non-syndromic craniosynostosis? A review of case-control studies. *J Oral Biol Craniofac Res,* 11, 78-83.

39. Carmichael SL, Ma C, Rasmussen SA, et al. (2008) Craniosynostosis and mater-nal smoking. *Birth Defects Res A Clin Mol Teratol,* 82, 78-85.

40. Sergesketter AR, Elsamadicy AA, Lubkin DT, et al. (2019) Characterization of perinatal risk factors and complications associated with nonsyndromic cranio-synostosis. *J Craniofac Surg,* 30, 334-338.

41. Rasmussen SA, Yazdy MM, Carmichael SL, et al. (2007) Maternal thyroid disease as a risk factor for craniosynostosis. *Obstet Gynecol,* 110, 369-77.

42. Carmichael SL, Ma C, Rasmussen SA, et al. (2015) Craniosynostosis and risk factors related to thyroid dysfunction. *Am J Med Genet A,* 167A, 701-7.

43. Berard A, Zhao JP, Sheehy O (2015) Sertraline use during pregnancy and the risk of major malformations. *Am J Obstet Gynecol,* 212, 795 1-12.

44. Lajeunie E, Barcik U, Thorne JA, et al. (2001) Craniosynostosis and fetal exposure to sodium valproate. *J Neurosurg,* 95, 778-82.

45. Plakas S, Anagnostou E, Plakas AC, Piagkou M (2022) High risk factors for craniosynostosis during pregnancy: A case-control study. *Eur J Obstet Gynecol Reprod Biol X,* 14, 1-5.

46. Tahiri Y, Bartlett SP, Gilardino MS (2017) Evidence-based medicine: Nonsyndro-mic craniosynostosis. *Plast Reconstr Surg,* 140, 177-191.

47. Piña-Garza JE, James KC (2019) *Fenichel's clinical pediatric neurology.* Philadelphia: Elsevier Health Sciences.

48. Birgfeld CB, Saltzman BS, Hing AV, et al. (2013) Making the diagnosis: Metopic ridge versus metopic craniosynostosis. *J Craniofac Surg,* 24, 178-85.

49. Fine A, Schupack K, Nickels K, Youssef P, Schupack K (2022) Childhood neurologic conditions: Neuroanatomic abnormalities. In: Rew KT, editor, *FP essentials.* 523 ed. Leawood, KS, USA: American Academy of Family Physicians, pp 27-42.

50. Miller C, Losken HW, Towbin R, et al. (2002) Ultrasound diagnosis of cranio-synostosis. *Cleft Palate Craniofac J,* 39, 73-80.

51. Stanton E, Urata M, Chen JF, Chai Y (2022) The clinical manifestations, molecular mechanisms and treatment of craniosynostosis. *Dis Model Mech*, 15, 1-18.

52. Defreitas CA, Carr SR, Merck DL, et al. (2022) Prenatal diagnosis of craniosynostosis using ultrasound. *Plast Reconstr Surg*, 150, 1084-1089.

53. Sgouros S (2005) Skull vault growth in craniosynostosis. *Childs Nerv Syst*, 21, 861-70.

54. Duan M, Skoch J, Pan BS, Shah V (2021) Neuro-ophthalmological manifestations of craniosynostosis: Current perspectives. *Eye Brain*, 13, 29-40.

55. World Health Organization (2024) *Head circumference for age.* [online] Available at: <https://www.who.int/tools/child-growth-standards/standards/head-circumference-for-age> [Accessed April 2 2024].

56. Goetzinger M, Verius M, Eder R, Laimer I, Rasse M (2022) Retrospective investigation of cranial volume and cephalic index in patients with nonsyndromic sagittal synostosis operated by total vault remodeling. *Pediatr Neurosurg*, 57, 260-269.

57. Abdullah KA, Reed W (2018) 3D printing in medical imaging and healthcare services. *J Med Radiat Sci*, 65, 237-239.

58. National Institute of Biomedical Imaging and Bioengineering (2024) *Ultrasound.* [online] Available at: <https://www.nibib.nih.gov/science-education/science-topics/ultrasound> [Accessed January 19 2024].

59. Huff JS, Murr N (2023) *Seizure.* [e-book] Treasure Island, StatPearls Publishing. Available at: <https://www.ncbi.nlm.nih.gov/books/NBK430765/> [Accessed February 9 2024].

60. Kiriakopoulos E (2019) *Understanding seizures.* [online] Available at: <https://www.epilepsy.com/what-is-epilepsy/understanding-seizures> [Accessed February 9 2024].

61. Derderian C, Seaward J (2012) Syndromic craniosynostosis. *Semin Plast Surg*, 26, 64-75.

62. Xue AS, Buchanan EP, Hollier LH, Jr. (2022) Update in management of craniosynostosis. *Plast Reconstr Surg*, 149, 1209-1223.

63. Touzé R, Bremond-Gignac D, Robert MP (2019) Ophthalmological management in craniosynostosis. *Neurochirurgie*, 65, 310-317.

64. Bellaire CP, Devarajan A, Napoli JG, et al. (2022) Craniofacial dysmorphology in infants with non-syndromic unilateral coronal craniosynostosis. *J Craniofac Surg*, 33, 1903-1908.

65. National Eye Institute (2024) *Amblyopia (lazy eye).* [online] Available at: <https://www.nei.nih.gov/learn-about-eye-health/eye-conditions-and-diseases/amblyopia-lazy-eye> [Accessed January 19 2024].

66. Strahle J, Muraszko KM, Buchman SR, et al. (2011) Chiari malformation associated with craniosynostosis. *Neurosurg Focus*, 31, 1-8.

67. Fearon JA, Dimas V, Ditthakasem K (2016) Lambdoid craniosynostosis: The relationship with Chiari deformations and an analysis of surgical outcomes. *Plast Reconstr Surg*, 137, 946-951.

68. Botelho RV, Botelho PB, Hernandez B, Sales MB, Rotta JM (2021) Association between brachycephaly, Chiari malformation, and basilar invagination. *J Neurol Surg A Cent Eur Neurosurg*, 84, 329-333.

69. Dhakal A, Bobrin BD (2023) *Cognitive deficits.* [e-book] Treasure Island (FL), StatPearls Publishing. Available at: National Library of Medicine <https://www .ncbi.nlm.nih.gov/books/NBK559052/> [Accessed January 30 2024].

70. Sackett DL, Rosenberg WM, Gray JA, Haynes RB, Richardson WS (1996) Evidence based medicine: What it is and what it isn't. *BMJ,* 312, 71-2.

71. Siminoff LA (2013) Incorporating patient and family preferences into evidence-based medicine. *BMC Med Inform Decis Mak,* 13, 1-7.

72. Agency for Healthcare Research and Quality (2020) *The share approach: A model for shared decisionmaking - fact sheet.* [online] Available at: <https:// www.ahrq.gov/health-literacy/professional-training/shared-decision/tools/fact sheet.html> [Accessed January 19 2024].

73. Gallagher ER, Fulton GK, Susarla SM, Birgfeld CB (2022) Multidisciplinary care considerations for patients with craniosynostosis. *Oral Maxillofac Surg Clin North Am,* 34, 353-365.

74. Badiee RK, Maru J, Yang SC, et al. (2022) Racial and socioeconomic disparities in prompt craniosynostosis workup and treatment. *J Craniofac Surg,* 33, 2422-2426.

75. Hoffman C, Valenti A, Buontempo M, Imahiyerobo T (2022) A retrospective analysis of the impact of health disparities on treatment for single suture cranio-synostosis before and during the pandemic. *Cleft Palate Craniofac J,* 1-8.

76. Lin Y, Pan IW, Harris DA, Luerssen TG, Lam S (2015) The impact of insurance, race, and ethnicity on age at surgical intervention among children with nonsyn-dromic craniosynostosis. *J Pediatr,* 166, 1289-96.

77. Vinchon M (2019) What remains of non-syndromic bicoronal synostosis? *Neurochirurgie,* 65, 252-257.

78. Borad V, Cordes EJ, Liljeberg KM, et al. (2019) Isolated lambdoid craniosyn-ostosis. *J Craniofac Surg,* 30, 2390-2392.

79. Reardon T, Fiani B, Kosarchuk J, Parisi A, Shlobin NA (2022) Management of lambdoid craniosynostosis: A comprehensive and systematic review. *Pediatr Neurosurg,* 57, 1-16.

80. Starr JR, Collett BR, Gaither R, et al. (2012) Multicenter study of neurodevel-opment in 3-year-old children with and without single-suture craniosynostosis. *Arch Pediatr Adolesc Med,* 166, 536-42.

81. Speltz ML, Collett BR, Wallace ER, et al. (2015) Intellectual and academic functioning of school-age children with single-suture craniosynostosis. *Pediatrics,* 135, 615-23.

82. American Psychological Association (2018) *APA dictionary of psychology.* [online] Available at: <https://dictionary.apa.org/> [Accessed January 19 2024].

83. American Psychiatric Association (2022) *Diagnostic and statistical man-ual of mental disorders: DSM-5.* Washington, DC: American Psychiatric Association Publishing.

84. Junn AH, Long AS, Hauc SC, et al. (2023a) Long-term neurocognitive outcomes in 204 single-suture craniosynostosis patients. *Childs Nerv Syst,* 1, 1-8.

85. Bellew M, Chumas P (2015) Long-term developmental follow-up in children with nonsyndromic craniosynostosis. *J Neurosurg Pediatr,* 16, 445-51.

86. Patel A, Yang JF, Hashim PW, et al. (2014) The impact of age at surgery on long-term neuropsychological outcomes in sagittal craniosynostosis. *Plast Reconstr Surg,* 134, 608-617.

87. American Psychological Association (2008) *Clinical neuropsychology.* [online] Available at: <https://www.apa.org/ed/graduate/specialize/neuropsychology> [Accessed January 19 2024].

88. Tandon D, Skolnick GB, Naidoo SD, et al. (2021) Morphologic severity of craniosynostosis: Implications for speech and neurodevelopment. *Cleft Palate Craniofac J,* 58, 1361-1369.

89. Naran S, Miller M, Shakir S, et al. (2017) Nonsyndromic craniosynostosis and associated abnormal speech and language development. *Plast Reconstr Surg,* 140, 62-69.

90. Goh LC, Azman A, Siti HBK, et al. (2018) An audiological evaluation of syndromic and non-syndromic craniosynostosis in pre-school going children. *Int J Pediatr Otorhinolaryngol,* 109, 50-53.

91. Lieu JEC, Kenna M, Anne S, Davidson L (2020) Hearing loss in children: A review. *Jama,* 324, 2195-2205.

92. Wenger TL, Hing AV, Evans KN (2019) Apert syndrome. In: Adam MP, Feldman J, Mirzaa GM, et al. editors, *GeneReviews.* Seattle: University of Washington.

93. O'hara J, Ruggiero F, Wilson L, et al. (2019) Syndromic craniosynostosis: Complexities of clinical care. *Mol Syndromol,* 10, 83-97.

94. Breik O, Mahindu A, Moore MH, et al. (2016) Central nervous system and cervical spine abnormalities in Apert syndrome. *Childs Nerv Syst,* 32, 833-8.

95. Munarriz PM, Pascual B, Castano-Leon AM, et al. (2020) Apert syndrome: Cranial procedures and brain malformations in a series of patients. *Surg Neurol Int,* 11, 1-8.

96. Casteleyn T, Horn D, Henrich W, Verlohren S (2022) Differential diagnosis of syndromic craniosynostosis: A case series. *Arch Gynecol Obstet,* 306, 49-57.

97. Udayakumaran S, Krishnadas A, Subash P (2022) Multisuture and syndromic craniosynostoses: Simplifying the complex. *J Pediatr Neurosci,* 17, 29-43.

98. Cohen MM (2011) Apert, Crouzon, and Pfeiffer syndromes. In: Muenke M, Kress W, Collmann H, Solomon B, editors, *Craniosynostoses: Molecular genetics, principles of diagnosis and treatment.* Halifax: Karger, pp 67-88.

99. Bartlett SP, Derderian CA (2014) Craniosynostosis syndromes. In: Thorne CH, editor, *Grabb and Smith's plastic surgery.* 7th ed. Philadelphia: Wolters Kluwer, pp 232-240.

100. Raam MS (2011) Uncommon craniosynostosis syndromes: A review of thirteen conditions. In: Muenke M, Kress W, Collmann H, Solomon B, editors, *Craniosynostoses: Molecular genetics, principles of diagnosis and treatment.* Bethesda: Karger, pp 119-142.

101. Wenger T, Miller D, Evans K (2020) FGFR craniosynostosis syndromes overview. In: Adam MP, Feldman J, Mirzaa GM, et al., editors, *GeneReviews.* Seattle: University of Washington.

102. Fearon JA, Rhodes J (2009) Pfeiffer syndrome: A treatment evaluation. *Plast Reconstr Surg,* 123, 1560-1569.

103. Das JM, Winters R (2023) *Pfeiffer syndrome*. [e-book] Treasure Island (FL), StatPearls Publishing, Available at: National Library of Medicine <https://www.ncbi.nlm.nih.gov/books/NBK532882/> [Accessed March 29 2024].

104. Mavridis IN, Rodrigues D (2021) Nervous system involvement in Pfeiffer syndrome. *Childs Nerv Syst*, 37, 367-374.

105. Reardon W, Winter RM (1994) Saethre-Chotzen syndrome. *J Med Genet*, 31, 393-6.

106. Gallagher ER, Ratisoontorn C, Cunningham ML (2019) Saethre-Chotzen syndrome. In: Adam MP, Feldman J, Mirzaa GM, et al. editors, *GeneReviews*. Seattle: University of Washington.

107. Alam MK, Alfawzan AA, Srivastava KC, et al. (2022) Craniofacial morphology in Apert syndrome: A systematic review and meta-analysis. *Sci Rep*, 12, 5708.

108. Conrady CD, Patel BC (2023) *Crouzon syndrome*. [e-book] Treasure Island (FL), StatPearls Publishing. Available at: National Library of Medicine <https://www.ncbi.nlm.nih.gov/books/NBK518998/> [Accessed March 29 2024].

109. Kruszka P, Rolle M, Kahle KT, Muenke M (2023) Muenke syndrome. In: Adam MP, Feldman J, Mirzaa GM, et al., editors, *GeneReviews*. Seattle: University of Washington.

110. Dicus Brookes C, Golden BA, Turvey TA (2014) Craniosynostosis syndromes. *Atlas Oral Maxillofac Surg Clin North Am*, 22, 103-10.

111. National Human Genome Research Institute (2018) *Genetics vs. Genomics fact sheet*. [online] Available at: <https://www.genome.gov/about-genomics/fact-sheets/Genetics-vs-Genomics> [Accessed March 28 2024].

112. Centers for Disease Control and Prevention (2022) *Genetic testing*. [online] Available at: <https://www.cdc.gov/genomics/gtesting/genetic_testing.htm> [Accessed March 28 2024].

113. Kimonis V, Gold JA, Hoffman TL, Panchal J, Boyadjiev SA (2007) Genetics of craniosynostosis. *Semin Pediatr Neurol*, 14, 150-61.

114. Johnson D, Wilkie AO (2011) Craniosynostosis. *Eur J Hum Genet*, 19, 369-76.

115. Ko JM (2016) Genetic syndromes associated with craniosynostosis. *J Korean Neurosurg Soc*, 59, 187-91.

116. Alam MK, Alfawzan AA, Abutayyem H, et al. (2023) Craniofacial characteristics in Crouzon's syndrome: A systematic review and meta-analysis. *Sci Prog*, 106, 368504231156297.

117. Tripathi T, Srivastava D, Bhutiani N, Rai P (2022) Comprehensive management of Crouzon syndrome: A case report with three-year follow-up. *J Orthod*, 49, 71-78.

118. Vogels A, Fryns JP (2006) Pfeiffer syndrome. *Orphanet J Rare Dis*, 1, 19-21.

119. Pelc A, Mikulewicz M (2018) Saethre-Chotzen syndrome: Case report and literature review. *Dent Med Probl*, 55, 217-225.

120. Abulezz TA, Allam KA, Wan DC, Lee JC, Kawamoto HK (2020) Saethre-Chotzen syndrome: A report of 7 patients and review of the literature. *Ann Plast Surg*, 85, 251-255.

121. Shakir S, Birgfeld CB (2022) Syndromic craniosynostosis: Cranial vault expansion in infancy. *Oral Maxillofac Surg Clin North Am*, 34, 443-458.

122. Sawh-Martinez R, Steinbacher DM (2019) Syndromic craniosynostosis. *Clin Plast Surg*, 46, 141-155.

123. Manjila S, Chim H, Eisele S, et al. (2010) History of the Kleeblattschädel deformity: Origin of concepts and evolution of management in the past 50 years. *Neurosurg Focus*, 29, 1-8.

124. Kalmar CL, Zapatero ZD, Kosyk MS, et al. (2021) Elevated intracranial pressure with craniosynostosis: A multivariate model of age, syndromic status, and number of involved cranial sutures. *J Neurosurg Pediatr*, 28, 716-723.

125. Kruszka P, Addissie YA, Yarnell CM, et al. (2016) Muenke syndrome: An international multicenter natural history study. *Am J Med Genet A*, 170a, 918-29.

126. Bonfield CM, Shannon CN, Reeder RW, et al. (2021) Hydrocephalus treatment in patients with craniosynostosis: An analysis from the hydrocephalus clinical research network prospective registry. *Neurosurg Focus*, 50, 1-7.

127. Frassanito P, Palombi D, Tamburrini G (2021) Craniosynostosis and hydrocephalus: Relevance and treatment modalities. *Childs Nerv Syst*, 37, 3465-3473.

128. Mathijssen IMJ, Working Group Guideline C (2021) Updated guideline on treatment and management of craniosynostosis. *J Craniofac Surg*, 32, 371-450.

129. Murali CN, McDonald-McGinn DM, Wenger TL, et al. (2019) Muenke syndrome: Medical and surgical comorbidities and long-term management. *Am J Med Genet A*, 179, 1442-1450.

130. Den Ottelander BK, Van Veelen MC, De Goederen R, et al. (2021) Saethre-Chotzen syndrome: Long-term outcome of a syndrome-specific management protocol. *Dev Med Child Neurol*, 63, 104-110.

131. Agochukwu NB, Solomon BD, Muenke M (2014) Hearing loss in syndromic craniosynostoses: Otologic manifestations and clinical findings. *Int J Pediatr Otorhinolaryngol*, 78, 2037-47.

132. American Speech-Language-Hearing Association (2024) *Sensorineural hearing loss*. [online] Available at: <https://www.asha.org/public/hearing/Sensorineural-Hearing-Loss/> [Accessed February 9 2024].

133. Fadda MT, Ierardo G, Ladniak B, et al. (2015) Treatment timing and multidisciplinary approach in Apert syndrome. *Ann Stomatol (Roma)*, 6, 58-63.

134. Taylor JA, Bartlett SP (2017) What's new in syndromic craniosynostosis surgery? *Plast Reconstr Surg*, 140, 82-93.

135. Droubi L, Laflouf M, Tolibah YA, Comisi JC (2022) Apert syndrome: Dental management considerations and objectives. *J Oral Biol Craniofac Res*, 12, 370-375.

136. Kreiborg S, Cohen MM, Jr. (1992) The oral manifestations of Apert syndrome. *J Craniofac Genet Dev Biol*, 12, 41-8.

137. Bhattacharjee K, Rehman O, Venkatraman V, et al. (2022) Crouzon syndrome and the eye: An overview. *Indian J Ophthalmol*, 70, 2346-2354.

138. Choi TM, Kramer GJC, Goos JAC, et al. (2022) Evaluation of dental maturity in Muenke syndrome, Saethre-Chotzen syndrome, and TCF12-related craniosynostosis. *Eur J Orthod*, 44, 287-293.

139. Blount JP, Louis RG, Jr., Tubbs RS, Grant JH (2007) Pansynostosis: A review. *Childs Nerv Syst*, 23, 1103-9.

140. National Center for Advancing Translational Studies (2024a) *Pfeiffer syndrome.* [online] Available at: <https://rarediseases.info.nih.gov/diseases/7380/pfeiffer -syndrome> [Accessed January 19 2024].

141. Junn A, Dinis J, Lu X, et al. (2021) Facial dysmorphology in Saethre-Chotzen syndrome. *J Craniofac Surg*, 32, 2660-2665.

142. Choi TM, Lijten OW, Mathijssen IMJ, Wolvius EB, Ongkosuwito EM (2022) Craniofacial morphology and growth in Muenke syndrome, Saethre-Chotzen syndrome, and TCF12-related craniosynostosis. *Clin Oral Investig,* 26, 2927-2936.

143. Kress W, Collmann H (2011) Saethre-Chotzen syndrome: Clinical and molecular genetic aspects. In: Muenke M, Kress W, Collmann H, Solomon B, editors, *Craniosynostoses: Molecular genetics, principles of diagnosis and treatment.* Würzburg: Karger, pp 98-106.

144. American Heart Association (2024a) *Coarctation of the aorta (COA).* [online] Available at: <https://www.heart.org/en/health-topics/congenital-heart-defects /about-congenital-heart-defects/coarctation-of-the-aorta-coa> [Accessed February 9 2024].

145. American Heart Association (2024b) *Patent ductus arteriosus (PDA).* [online] Available at: <https://www.heart.org/en/health-topics/congenital-heart-defects /about-congenital-heart-defects/patent-ductus-arteriosus-pda> [Accessed February 9 2024].

146. Solomon BD, Muenke M (2011) Muenke syndrome. In: Muenke M, Kress W, Collmann H, Solomon B, editors, *Craniosynostoses: Molecular genetics, principles of diagnosis and treatment.* Bethesda: Karger, pp 89-97.

147. National Center for Advancing Translational Studies (2024b) *Saethre-Chotzen syndrome.* [online] Available at: <https://rarediseases.info.nih.gov/diseases/7598 /saethre-chotzen-syndrome> [Accessed January 19 2024].

148. Mathews F, Shaffer AD, Georg MW, et al. (2019) Airway anomalies in patients with craniosynostosis. *Laryngoscope*, 129, 2594-2602.

149. Bohm LA, Sidman JD, Roby B (2016) Early airway intervention for craniofacial anomalies. *Facial Plast Surg Clin North Am*, 24, 427-436.

150. Yang S, Mathijssen IMJ, Joosten KFM (2022) The impact of obstructive sleep apnea on growth in patients with syndromic and complex craniosynostosis: A retrospective study. *Eur J Pediatr*, 181, 4191-4197.

151. Pickrell BB, Meaike JD, Canadas KT, Chandy BM, Buchanan EP (2017) Tracheal cartilaginous sleeve in syndromic craniosynostosis: An underrecognized source of significant morbidity and mortality. *J Craniofac Surg*, 28, 696-699.

152. Buchanan EP, Xue Y, Xue AS, Olshinka A, Lam S (2017) Multidisciplinary care of craniosynostosis. *J Multidiscip Healthc*, 10, 263-270.

153. McCarthy JG, Warren SM, Bernstein J, et al. (2012) Parameters of care for craniosynostosis. *Cleft Palate Craniofac J*, 49 Suppl, 23.

154. Jamieson NC, Tadi P (2023) *Feeding tube.* [e-book] Treasure Island (FL), StatPearls Publishing. Available at: National Library of Medicine <https://www .ncbi.nlm.nih.gov/books/NBK559044/> [Accessed March 29 2024].

155. Saad M (2019) Defining and determining intellectual disability insights from DSM-5. *International journal of Psycho-Educational Sciences*, 8, 51-54.

156. Maliepaard M, Mathijssen IM, Oosterlaan J, Okkerse JM (2014) Intellectual, behavioral, and emotional functioning in children with syndromic craniosynostosis. *Pediatrics*, 133, 1608-15.

157. American Society of Anesthesiologists (2024) *What does an anesthesiologist do?* [online] Available at: <https://asahq.org/madeforthismoment/anesthesia-101/role -of-physician-anesthesiologist/> [Accessed January 19 2024].

158. Clayman MA, Murad GJ, Steele MH, Seagle MB, Pincus DW (2007) History of craniosynostosis surgery and the evolution of minimally invasive endoscopic techniques: The University of Florida experience. *Ann Plast Surg*, 58, 285-7.

159. Holley TJ, Ranalli NJ, Steinberg B (2022) Historical perspectives on the management of craniosynostosis. *Oral and Maxillofacial Surgery Clinics of North America*, 34, 333-340.

160. Bruce WJ, Chang V, Joyce CJ, et al. (2018) Age at time of craniosynostosis repair predicts increased complication rate. *Cleft Palate Craniofac J*, 55, 649 654.

161. Koppel D, Grant J (2021) Modern management of craniosynostosis. In: Bonanthaya K, Panneerselvam E, Manuel S, Kumar VV, Rai A, editors, *Oral and maxillofacial surgery for the clinician*. Singapore: Springer, pp 1813-1841.

162. Bennett KG, Hespe GE, Vercler CJ, Buchman SR (2019) Short- and long-term outcomes by procedure type for nonsagittal single-suture craniosynostosis. *J Craniofac Surg*, 30, 458-464.

163. Ha AY, Skolnick GB, Chi D, et al. (2020) School-aged anthropometric outcomes after endoscopic or open repair of metopic synostosis. *Pediatrics*, 146.

164. Puthumana JS, Lopez CD, Lake IV, Yang R (2023) Evaluation of complications and outcomes in craniosynostosis by age of operation: Analysis of the national surgical quality improvement program-pediatric. *J Craniofac Surg*, 34, 29-33.

165. Yan H, Abel TJ, Alotaibi NM, et al. (2018a) A systematic review and meta-analysis of endoscopic versus open treatment of craniosynostosis. Part 1: The sagittal suture. *J Neurosurg Pediatr*, 22, 352-360.

166. Yan H, Abel TJ, Alotaibi NM, et al. (2018b) A systematic review of endoscopic versus open treatment of craniosynostosis. Part 2: The nonsagittal single sutures. *J Neurosurg Pediatr*, 22, 361-368.

167. Rizvi I, Harrison LM, Parsa S, et al. (2022) Open versus minimally invasive approach for craniosynostosis: Analysis of the national surgical quality improvement program-pediatric. *Cleft Palate Craniofac J*, 1-6.

168. Mundinger GS, Rehim SA, Johnson O, 3rd, et al. (2016) Distraction osteogenesis for surgical treatment of craniosynostosis: A systematic review. *Plast Reconstr Surg*, 138, 657-669.

169. Coombs DM, Knackstedt R, Patel N (2022) Optimizing blood loss and management in craniosynostosis surgery: A systematic review of outcomes over the last 40 years. *Cleft Palate Craniofac J*, 1-13.

170. Persing JA (2008) MOC-PS(SM) CME article: Management considerations in the treatment of craniosynostosis. *Plast Reconstr Surg*, 121, 1-11.

171. Menon G, George M, Kumar P, et al. (2022) Comparison of perioperative anesthetic concerns in simple and complex craniosynostosis cases: A retrospective study. *J Neuroanaesth Crit Care*, 09, 029-034.

172. Lai LL, See MH, Rampal S, Ng KS, Chan L (2019) Significant factors influencing inadvertent hypothermia in pediatric anesthesia. *J Clin Monit Comput*, 33, 1105-1112.

173. Thomas K, Hughes C, Johnson D, Das S (2012) Anesthesia for surgery related to craniosynostosis: A review. Part 1. *Paediatr Anaesth*, 22, 1033-41.

174. Chumble A, Brush P, Muzaffar A, Tanaka T (2022) The effects of preoperative administration of erythropoietin in pediatric patients undergoing cranial vault remodeling for craniosynostosis. *J Craniofac Surg*, 33, 1424-1427.

175. Wood RJ, Stewart CN, Liljeberg K, Sylvanus TS, Lim PK (2020) Transfusion-free cranial vault remodeling: A novel, multifaceted approach. *Plast Reconstr Surg*, 145, 167-174.

176. Zheng XQ, Huang JF, Lin JL, Chen D, Wu AM (2020) Effects of preoperative warming on the occurrence of surgical site infection: A systematic review and meta-analysis. *Int J Surg*, 77, 40-47.

177. Solutions for Patient Safety (2024) *Additional HAC resources*. [online] Available at: <https://www.solutionsforpatientsafety.org/hac-resources> [Accessed January 19 2024].

178. Kadakia S, Badhey A, Ashai S, Lee TS, Ducic Y (2017) Alopecia following bicoronal incisions. *JAMA Facial Plast Surg*, 19, 220-224.

179. Manworren RC, Stinson J (2016) Pediatric pain measurement, assessment, and evaluation. *Semin Pediatr Neurol*, 23, 189-200.

180. Gillette Children's (2024) *Recovery from surgery*. [online] Available at: <https://www.gillettechildrens.org/your-visit/prepare-for-your-visit/prepare-for-surgery/recovery-from-surgery> [Accessed February 9 2024].

181. Brand K, Al-Rais A (2019) Pain assessment in children. *Anaesthesia & Intensive Care Medicine*, 20, 314-317.

182. Mortada H, Alkhashan R, Alhindi N, et al. (2022) The management of perioperative pain in craniosynostosis repair: A systematic literature review of the current practices and guidelines for the future. *Maxillofac Plast Reconstr Surg*, 44:33, 1-18.

183. Wood RJ (2012) Craniosynostosis and deformational plagiocephaly: When and how to intervene. *Minn Med*, 95, 46-9.

184. Kim SY, Park MS, Yang JI, Yim SY (2013) Comparison of helmet therapy and counter positioning for deformational plagiocephaly. *Ann Rehabil Med*, 37, 785-95.

185. Robinson S, Proctor M (2009) Diagnosis and management of deformational plagiocephaly. *J Neurosurg Pediatr*, 3, 284-95.

186. Kaplan SL, Coulter C, Sargent B (2018) Physical therapy management of congenital muscular torticollis: A 2018 evidence-based clinical practice guideline from the APTA Academy of Pediatric Physical Therapy. *Pediatr Phys Ther*, 30, 240-290.

187. Jullien S (2021) Sudden infant death syndrome prevention. *BMC Pediatr*, 21, 1-9.

188. Di Chiara A, La Rosa E, Ramieri V, Vellone V, Cascone P (2019) Treatment of deformational plagiocephaly with physiotherapy. *J Craniofac Surg*, 30, 2008-2013.

189. Task Force on Infant Sleep Position and Sudden Infant Death Syndrome (2000) Changing concepts of sudden infant death syndrome: Implications for infant sleeping environment and sleep position. *Pediatrics, 105,* 650-6.

190. Turk AE, McCarthy JG, Thorne CH, Wisoff JH (1996) The "back to sleep campaign" and deformational plagiocephaly: Is there cause for concern? *J Craniofac Surg, 7,* 12-8.

191. Van Cruchten C, Feijen MMW, Van Der Hulst R (2021) Demographics of positional plagiocephaly and brachycephaly; risk factors and treatment. *J Craniofac Surg, 32,* 2736-2740.

192. Santiago GS, Santiago CN, Chwa ES, Purnell CA (2023) Positional plagiocephaly and craniosynostosis. *Pediatr Ann, 52,* 10-17.

193. Roby BB, Finkelstein M, Tibesar RJ, Sidman JD (2012) Prevalence of positional plagiocephaly in teens born after the "back to sleep" campaign. *Otolaryngol Head Neck Surg, 146,* 823-8.

194. Ditthakasem K, Kolar JC (2017) Deformational plagiocephaly: A review. *Pediatr Nurs, 43,* 59-64.

195. Kunz F, Schweitzer T, Dörr A, et al. (2020) Craniofacial growth in infants with deformational plagiocephaly: Does prematurity affect the duration of head orthosis therapy and the extent of the reduction in asymmetry during treatment? *Clin Oral Investig, 24,* 2991-2999.

196. Fabre-Grenet M, Garcia-Méric P, Bernard-Niel V, et al. (2017) Effects of deformational plagiocephaly during the first 12 months on the psychomotor development of prematurely born infants. *Arch Pediatr, 24,* 802-810.

197. De Bock F, Braun V, Renz-Polster H (2017) Deformational plagiocephaly in normal infants: A systematic review of causes and hypotheses. *Arch Dis Child, 102,* 535-542.

198. Nuysink J, Van Haastert IC, Eijsermans MJ, et al. (2012) Prevalence and predictors of idiopathic asymmetry in infants born preterm. *Early Hum Dev, 88,* 387-92.

199. Gross PW, Chipman DE, Doyle SM (2023) The tilts, twists, and turns of torticollis. *Curr Opin Pediatr, 35,* 118-123.

200. Rogers GF, Oh AK, Mulliken JB (2009) The role of congenital muscular torticollis in the development of deformational plagiocephaly. *Plast Reconstr Surg, 123,* 643-652.

201. Trottier N, Hurtubise K, Camden C, Cloutier W, Gaboury I (2023) Barriers and facilitators influencing parental adherence to prevention strategies for deformational plagiocephaly: Results from a scoping review. *Child Care Health Dev, 49,* 852-869.

202. Özkılıç A, Çevik S, Isik S (2020) The role of age on effectiveness of active repositioning therapy in positional skull deformities. *The Journal of Basic and Clinical Health Sciences, 1,* 33-37.

203. Collett B, Breiger D, King D, Cunningham M, Speltz M (2005) Neurodevelopmental implications of "deformational" plagiocephaly. *J Dev Behav Pediatr, 26,* 379-89.

204. Hewitt L, Kerr E, Stanley RM, Okely AD (2020) Tummy time and infant health outcomes: A systematic review. *Pediatrics, 145.*

205. World Health Organization (2019) *New WHO guidelines on physical activity, sedentary behaviour and sleep for children under 5 years of age.* [online] Available at: <https://www.who.int/news/item/24-04-2019-to-grow-up-healthy -children-need-to-sit-less-and-play-more> [Accessed January 19 2024].

206. Kuo AA, Tritasavit S, Graham JM, Jr. (2014) Congenital muscular torticollis and positional plagiocephaly. *Pediatr Rev,* 35, 79-87.

207. Cabrera-Martos I, Valenza MC, Benítez-Feliponi A, et al. (2013) Clinical profile and evolution of infants with deformational plagiocephaly included in a conservative treatment program. *Childs Nerv Syst,* 29, 1893-8.

208. American Academy of Pediatrics (2021) *Movement milestones: Babies 4 to 7 months.* [online] Available at: <https://www.healthychildren.org/English/ages -stages/baby/Pages/Movement-4-to-7-Months.aspx> [Accessed January 19 2024].

209. Tamber MS, Nikas D, Beier A, et al. (2016) Congress of neurological surgeons systematic review and evidence-based guideline on the role of cranial molding orthosis (helmet) therapy for patients with positional plagiocephaly. *Neurosurgery,* 79, 632-633.

210. Jung BK, Yun IS (2020) Diagnosis and treatment of positional plagiocephaly. *Arch Craniofac Surg,* 21, 80-86.

211. Clarren SK, Smith DW, Hanson JW (1979) Helmet treatment for plagiocephaly and congenital muscular torticollis. *J Pediatr,* 94, 43-6.

212. Goh JL, Bauer DF, Durham SR, Stotland MA (2013) Orthotic (helmet) therapy in the treatment of plagiocephaly. *Neurosurg Focus,* 35, 1-6.

213. Steinberg JP, Rawlani R, Humphries LS, Rawlani V, Vicari FA (2015) Effectiveness of conservative therapy and helmet therapy for positional cranial deformation. *Plast Reconstr Surg,* 135, 833-842.

214. Visse HS, Meyer U, Runte C, Maas H, Dirksen D (2020) Assessment of facial and cranial symmetry in infants with deformational plagiocephaly undergoing molding helmet therapy. *J Craniomaxillofac Surg,* 48, 548-554.

215. Park KM, Tripathi NV, Mufarrej FA (2021) Quality of life in patients with craniosynostosis and deformational plagiocephaly: A systematic review. *Int J Pediatr Otorhinolaryngol,* 149, 1-9.

216. Kunz F, Schweitzer T, Große S, et al. (2019) Head orthosis therapy in positional plagiocephaly: Longitudinal 3D-investigation of long-term outcomes, compared with untreated infants and with a control group. *Eur J Orthod,* 41, 29-37.

217. Junn A, Dinis J, Long A, et al. (2023b) Disparities in access to cranial remodeling orthosis for deformational plagiocephaly. *Cleft Palate Craniofac J,* 60, 454-460.

218. Pellicer E, Siebold BS, Birgfeld CB, Gallagher ER (2018) Evaluating trends in headache and revision surgery following cranial vault remodeling for craniosynostosis. *Plast Reconstr Surg,* 141, 725-734.

219. Rotimi O, Jung GP, Ong J, et al. (2021) Sporting activity after craniosynostosis surgery in children: A source of parental anxiety. *Childs Nerv Syst,* 37, 287-290.

220. Yengo-Kahn AM, Akinnusotu O, Wiseman AL, et al. (2021) Sport participation and related head injuries following craniosynostosis correction: A survey study. *Neurosurg Focus,* 50, 1-6.

221. Kljajic M, Maltese G, Tarnow P, Sand P, Kolby L (2023) Health-related quality of life of children treated for non-syndromic craniosynostosis. *J Plast Surg Hand Surg, 57,* 408-414.

222. Akai T, Yamashita M, Shiro T, et al. (2022) Long-term outcomes of non-syndromic and syndromic craniosynostosis: Analysis of demographic, morphologic, and surgical factors. *Neurol Med Chir (Tokyo), 62,* 57-64.

223. Baykal D, Balcin RN, Taskapilioglu MO (2022) Amount of reoperation following surgical repair of nonsyndromic craniosynostosis at a single center. *Turk J Med Sci, 52,* 1235-1240.

224. Klieverik VM, Singhal A, Woerdeman PA (2023) Cosmetic satisfaction and patient-reported outcomes following surgical treatment of single-suture cranio-synostosis: A systematic review. *Childs Nerv Syst, 39,* 3571-3581.

225. Rhodes G (2006) The evolutionary psychology of facial beauty. *Annu Rev Psychol, 57,* 199-226.

226. Azoulay-Avinoam S, Bruun R, Maclaine J, et al. (2020) An overview of cranio-synostosis craniofacial syndromes for combined orthodontic and surgical management. *Oral Maxillofac Surg Clin North Am, 32,* 233-247.

227. American Pregnancy Association (2024) *IVF - in vitro fertilization.* [online] Available at: <https://americanpregnancy.org/getting-pregnant/infertility/in-vitro-fertilization/> [Accessed January 19 2024].

228. Simon LV, Hashmi MF, Bragg BN (2023) *Apgar score.* [e-book] Treasure Island (FL), StatPearls Publishing. Available at: National Library of Medicine <https://www.ncbi.nlm.nih.gov/books/NBK542197/> [Accessed March 29 2024].

229. Academy of Pediatric Physical Therapy, (2019) Fact sheet: The ABCs of pediatric physical therapy. [pdf] Middleton WI, Academy of Pediatric Physical Therapy, Available at: <https://pediatricapta.org/includes/fact-sheets/pdfs/FactSheet_ABCs ofPediatricPT_2019.pdf?v=2> [Accessed April 24 2024].

Index

Abbreviations used in index: CS *craniosynostosis,* DP *deformational plagiocephaly. Figures and tables indicated by page numbers in italics.*